THE HEALING

WISDOM OF

DREAMS

THE HEALING WISDOM OF DREAMS

Discover Your True Self
through Lucid Dreaming,
Journalling and Visioning

Kathleen
Webster O'Malley

HAY HOUSE

Carlsbad, California • New York City
London • Sydney • New Delhi

Published in the United Kingdom by:
Hay House UK Ltd, The Sixth Floor, Watson House,
54 Baker Street, London W1U 7BU
Tel: +44 (0)20 3927 7290; Fax: +44 (0)20 3927 7291; www.hayhouse.co.uk

Published in the United States of America by:
Hay House Inc., PO Box 5100, Carlsbad, CA 92018-5100
Tel: (1) 760 431 7695 or (800) 654 5126
Fax: (1) 760 431 6948 or (800) 650 5115; www.hayhouse.com

Published in Australia by:
Hay House Australia Ltd, 18/36 Ralph St, Alexandria NSW 2015
Tel: (61) 2 9669 4299; Fax: (61) 2 9669 4144; www.hayhouse.com.au

Published in India by:
Hay House Publishers India, Muskaan Complex, Plot No.3, B-2,
Vasant Kunj, New Delhi 110 070
Tel: (91) 11 4176 1620; Fax: (91) 11 4176 1630; www.hayhouse.co.in

Project editor: Anna Cooperberg
Cover design: Leah Jacobs-Gordon
Interior design: Karim J. Garcia
Illustrations on page 215 and 218: courtesy of Andrei Verner

A catalogue record for this book is available from the British Library.

Tradepaper ISBN: 978-1-78817-827-3
E-book ISBN: 978-1-4019-6914-1
Audiobook ISBN: 978-1-4019-6915-8

Printed and bound by CPI Group (UK) Ltd, Croydon, CR0 4YY

To Virginia Harrigan-Hodge Webster,
my grandmother, who nurtured my essential
gifts of dreaming and compassion. And to
her mother, Mary Louisa Harrigan,
who brought her into being.

CONTENTS

INTRODUCTION

MY GRANDMOTHER'S WISDOM

In the summer of 1989, when I was 15, I dreamed of walking along a familiar beach when I noticed a crib. Inside the crib, there was a fish. When I told my grandmother of this dream, she said it meant that someone was pregnant. "Oh, because of the crib?" I questioned. She said, "No, because of the fish." I had no reason to doubt my grandmother's wisdom since she had given birth to nine children, though she never fully explained the message of the fish.

My grandmother was my primary caregiver from infancy until just before I turned five, when my mom resumed care of me. We lived in a small fishing village known as Island Harbour on the island of Anguilla, a British territory in the Caribbean Sea. My grandmother was small in stature, yet she had an enormous presence. When you received a hug from her, it was with her entire being. When she looked you over, it was as though her eyes penetrated your entire being, arriving all the way to your soul. Though she had a calm demeanor, everyone knew to never cross her, as she was known for her sharp tongue just as much as her bright smile.

Before sunrise until late afternoon, my grandmother spent her days cooking, planting, or harvesting, and tending to her chickens, pigs, goats, and sheep while my grandfather, a sailor and fisherman, was at sea. She knew the earth. She understood its cycles and its rhythms. She somehow knew the benefits of every plant that grew around her, while I was more fascinated by the lizards and the bugs, including the caterpillars that I would find in her bucket of freshly husked corn.

Even after it was decided that I would return to living with my mom on the island of Saint Thomas, I still spent every summer with my grandparents. Even without electricity and indoor plumbing, my best childhood memories were at their home gallivanting about the island, as my grandmother would say. My grandmother was the person who listened to my nighttime dreams. Often she would tell me what my dreams meant. Other times, she would respond with, "Child, did you forget to say your prayers last night?" And sometimes she would simply respond with a short "Hmm," her lips firmly pressed together as though to indicate that someday I would understand what she knew the meaning to be but was not yet ready to hear it. As I journeyed into motherhood, my grandmother's interpretation of fish proved to be true. Dreams of fish became the way my inner wisdom communicated each time new life was growing inside of me.

I have experienced nine pregnancies, including three unexplained premature births. We also had two unsuccessful attempts at gestational surrogacy. Our only surviving daughter had been our second pregnancy. Weeks before my pregnancy with her was confirmed, I dreamed of a fish swimming in the sky. I knew exactly when I had conceived because of this dream, or so I thought. On the day I started to experience signs of preterm labor, an ultra sound measured her to be just 28 weeks gestation, not 34 weeks by my calculation. Up until then, my pregnancy was being followed by a midwife. Other than mild spot ting at about eight weeks gestation, this pregnancy had been uneventful, so there were no early ultrasounds.

When I saw my midwife, Sue, the morning after labor started, she explained that it was too early in my preg nancy to safely deliver at home. She accompanied my husband and me to the hospital, where I received steroid injections to speed up lung development and medication to prevent further contractions. A second ultrasound was done, and the findings were the same. "You are not more than 28 weeks," my doctors insisted. I questioned myself. *How could I have been so wrong?* I listened as they explained that despite their best efforts to stop labor, they had been unsuccessful. My only option was to have an emergency C-section, and so my tiny—but healthy—baby girl was delivered at 10:38 that evening. As it turns out, she was 34 weeks after all, and arrived at 18 inches long and weighing four pounds, seven ounces. After just 10 days in the neo natal intensive care unit, she was released to come home. It was then that I started to pay even closer attention to my dreams, as it was my dream that had shown me the truth of my daughter's coming to be in the womb, and in this world.

Needless to say, my waking dream of having a water birth in the comfort of my own home was never realized. It felt like the most natural option, as I grew up surrounded by the sea. Despite a near drowning at age 13, I am still drawn to bodies of water. Our home in central Massachusetts is on a peninsula surrounded by a large pond, and one of my favorite New England states is Maine, where the mountains meet the sea.

"Go to the sea," my grandmother used to say. She believed that the sea was the cure for just about any ailment, physical or otherwise. She would send us off without a word of caution. My cousins, my siblings, and I would swim in the ocean, often without any adult supervision. She trusted we would be okay, and we were. If we were to speak now, I know she would say, "Child, you were never unattended. I asked the sea to watch over all of you. If ever you ventured too far, its waves would gently usher you closer to shore. And now, now I am the sea . . ."

Whenever I have been in a state of grief, my dreams have taken me to the sea, and there I have found healing. After the loss of our daughter Jade, a second spontaneous preterm delivery, I returned to that familiar dreamscape and somehow the memory of the crib had entered my current dream. This was the summer of 2006. My dreaming mind began to search the beach for the crib, thinking that my baby girl was inside. Believing the crib had been swept away, I ran into the sea. A tidal wave appeared and gently lifted me out of the water, carrying me until I woke up. I now see that tidal wave as an aspect of my deeper self, helping me to awaken and not lose sight of my other daughter, a then two-year-old who needed her mother. My belief is that our deeper self is always reorienting us toward life and toward greater purpose.

THE VALUE OF OUR DREAMS

My work as an integrative wellness practitioner has allowed me to see that unacknowledged and unprocessed emotions can create physical symptoms deep within tissues of the body. Dreams come not to *fix* us, but to encourage us to explore our inner lives and guide us through life's most difficult moments. They connect us to the hidden, most vulnerable pieces of ourselves, to our essential gifts, and to unitive purpose. They illuminate paths through the darkest of times, helping us uncover who we truly are and all that we might become.

"Trust your body," I often tell my patients and wellness clients. Pain and discomfort, disappointment and uncertainty, loss and grief often take us away from listening to and trusting the wisdom of the body, the wisdom inherent in nature and all forms of life. When we trust in the wisdom of our dreams, we are trusting in our deepest self and in something bigger than ourselves: the force of life that allows us to exist as we are, a sense of community and shared purpose, a connection to a higher power by whichever name we choose. Some of my patients and wellness clients have graciously agreed to allow the sharing of their dreams and healing experiences in this book. Most names have been changed for privacy.

Likewise, my more mystical experiences have shown me that dreams allow us to glimpse other realities beyond the physical while awakening us to new ways of being in this world and with each other. They say our grandmothers once carried us in their wombs; I believe we now carry them in ours. I can almost hear my own grandmother saying, *I am the sea. I am the grains of sand, the starfish, the seashells. Hear my laughter in yours. See my smile in your smile . . . I am always near, for I am love, eternally.*

Our dreams serve as a bridge between our conscious mind, our sensing body, and our deepest conscience. They are invitations to greater self-awareness.

Through stories and dream journal entries, *The Healing Wisdom of Dreams* illustrates how engaging with our nightly visions gives us a sense of direction, helping us to heal current heartbreak, past hurt, and even pre-birth trauma, where the messages received while inside the mother's womb continue to impact our lives though we are consciously unaware of them.

Dreams can also be playful, inspiring our creativity and allowing us to open to innovative ways of thinking and being in the world. Researchers at the University of California, Berkeley, found study participants to have a 15 to 35 percent greater capacity for problem-solving when awakened during REM-sleep dreaming than they had when they were fully awake. According to Matthew Walker, Ph.D.[1], director of the Center for Human Sleep Science, it is during dreaming sleep that our brains take preconceived knowledge and make connections that create solutions to "previously impenetrable problems."

ENGAGING WITH AND UNDERSTANDING OUR DREAMS

While I share my journey to newfound strength and full-circle healing, this book also contains dream journaling exercises, visualizations, and meditative practices to help you cultivate a greater sense of trust in the voice of your inner being and invoke the gifts of our maternal heritage—all that nurtures, supports, connects, and binds us beyond space and time.

The first part of this book goes beyond dream analysis and interpretation. It outlines a pathway to reclaiming the essence of who you are, deepening your understanding of your inner world, uncovering the voice of your innermost wisdom and your innate gifts. Though I attempt to express this guidance in a linear sequence, when it comes to our deeper consciousness, it is not easy to define an absolute beginning, middle, and end. See this as a framework for developing a practice that honors the wisdom of your dreams.

The first half of this book provides specific tools, like techniques for enhancing dream recall and dream journaling and how to ask our dreams for guidance through a process known to the ancient Greeks as *dream incubation*. You'll learn how to better understand dream messages as they relate to immediate life circumstances, how to effectively address what we consider to be nightmares by re-visioning these urgent dreams, and how to develop self-compassion as we examine the more vulnerable aspects of ourselves, allowing us to heal unwanted patterns and live more authentically. Finally, you'll understand how to engage with dreams as dream play and excavate our inner gifts.

The second part of *The Healing Wisdom of Dreams* is about the mystical aspect of our lives, allowing us to see that our waking life is also a dream—a construct of our beliefs, imaginings, and expectations, influenced also by the world of spirit. We consider how ordinary and "big" dreams inform and transform our lives. We explore visitations from ancestors, guides, and loved ones who have transitioned, and learn about animal archetypes that commonly appear in dreams across cultures. These dream characters and figures deepen our understanding of the world within us and the world around us. We'll look at lucid dreaming as a healing technique, explore Tibetan dream yoga practices, and finally consider our shared dream for collective healing.

While no one person is responsible for ending all the suffering in the world, each one of us can participate in the greater healing by beginning with our own lives. The process of healing is not about putting the same broken pieces back together. Rather, it is about reclaiming what is already within us that could never be broken—the essence of who we are as individuals and as interconnected parts of a greater whole. It is recognizing that while there are no simple answers to life's greatest problems, life is constantly showing us who we have the potential to be. *The Healing Wisdom of Dreams* provides essential practices to engage with one's nightly dreams and awaken a greater understanding of how our challenges lead us to heal, create, and serve in this intricate web of life.

Part I

RECLAIMING THE ESSENCE OF WHO YOU ARE

Chapter 1

KEEPING A RECORD
OF YOUR JOURNEY

The day after our daughter's burial, my husband and I, along with our toddler, headed to the mountains of New Hampshire. There is something about the mountains and the trees; they seem to understand grief. As my husband loaded up the last of our bags, a yellow-and-black swallowtail butterfly caught my attention. It fluttered and danced about my window and continued to do so until we started to pull out of the driveway. It was a quiet ride. We made one stop the entire trip, at a small rest area, and took turns waiting with our daughter while the other went inside.

As I stood outside the car at the rest area, I noticed another swallowtail flying about before landing on a nearby bush. I felt completely present, surrounded by my daughter's chatter, the warmth of the morning sun, a soft breeze, and the butterfly. For a moment, I felt a reprieve from the deep sadness. Soon after arriving at our condo in the town of Lincoln, I walked to a nearby river to journal. I sat and allowed quiet tears and my words to flow. I lifted my gaze and was surprised to see a third swallowtail fluttering by. It occurred to me that maybe this was our baby's way of letting us know that she was not too far away.

That night, back at the river's edge, my dreaming mind placed me on a tall cliff. It was stormy and the winds were powerful, and I was afraid. Just as I was about to fall, I heard my grandmother call to me, "Kattee." I answered yes and woke up. I got out of bed and wrote these words at 5:55 a.m. on June 18, 2006:

> *My dear child, you are never to journey through pain and deep sadness alone. Cry out loud so that the winds of grace can hear your call for comfort. Stomp, if you must, so that the ground beneath might rise up to hold you if ever you should begin to fall. Just as these stones in and along this riverbed, allow the sorrows and the longings of your heart to mold and polish, but not destroy the essence of you . . .*

That was almost 15 years ago. If it were not for my journals, I might not have been able to recall that dream. Why would I want to remember? Why would I keep a record of my more challenging moments and my most frightening dreams? Why would I encourage you to do the same?

Quite simply, when we see the beauty and grace in how far we have come, we can never deny where we have been. When we allow ourselves to remember, we honor all aspects of who we currently are, everything we have ever lived, and all who came before us.

WHY KEEP A DREAM JOURNAL?

No matter how reliable one's memory might be, we cannot always recall events precisely as they occurred, as they are deeply colored by emotion. Dreams are even more fragile than our memories. They can rapidly dissipate as soon as we get out of bed, leaving us with only a vague sense of something worth pondering. Unlike distant memories, lost dreams are difficult to recapture, though it is possible to hear or see something during the day that might spark spontaneous dream recall. If the message is an important one, know that it will be offered again in the form of a recurring dream.

The only way to ensure consistent dream recall is to keep a record of your dreams. Weeks later, you may struggle to remember even the most vivid dream. The practice of recording your dreams not only helps you to remember, but it also engages your deepest consciousness. It expresses your readiness to receive even more. With repetition, you gain a greater understanding of what lives in your deeper consciousness, and it allows you to tap into a potential that is just waiting to be expressed in your waking life. Journaling helps us look back and witness the beautiful unfolding of our dreams with greater perspective. It allows us to connect images and phrases from our dream states to synchronicities that arise throughout the day.

TRUSTING IN THE PRACTICE

For some, there is nothing scarier than putting your innermost thoughts to paper—it makes them real. Though this may be difficult, it has incredible value. Overcoming the fear is what will lead you to engage with your deeper wisdom, a source of unwavering guidance that reveals your innate gifts and all that you are. By allowing yourself to write down what has come up in your nightly visions, no matter how hard, you can access a reservoir of healing and connection. Yes, you may remember something from long ago that is painful, something you had hoped to forget. But this process allows you to live with greater authenticity and build a more solid, secure, compassionate sense of self.

Trust that your innermost being is wise and will bring to the surface only what you are truly ready to process. Know that your inner psyche waits patiently until you have just enough solidity and support in place. It will give you the space to decide consciously when to begin this transformative process of healing and growth. Once you begin, your dreams will give you the courage to continue along this path of self-knowledge to self-mastery.

THE LANGUAGE OF DREAMS

Dreams can be poetic in nature, showing us where to place our attention without telling us exactly what to see. Like the workings of a telegraph, our inner psyche transmits messages from the deepest parts of our bioelectrical bodies, our cells, our tissues, our unconscious mind, and our innermost being. Our dreams hold elements of our waking lives. They are keepers of both our most beautiful and most painful memories. They reveal what is ready to be acknowledged, processed, and healed. They also hold ancestral memories. While dreams are typically not meant to be taken literally, they should never be dismissed simply as remnants of our daily interactions or random electrochemical by-products of the brain—especially when we sense there is something more to be learned. And often this sense that there is something to explore is what leads us to feel apprehensive. Challenge this feeling and look inward.

Keeping a journal allows you to further reflect on themes and images that are most meaningful to you. For example, in November 2019 I had a dream in which I was handed a book by a male figure wearing a crimson robe who appeared to be of East Indian descent. As he offered me the book he spoke the words: "I give you *giok*." As I recalled my dream, I was curious about the fact that this dream figure used a word that was unfamiliar, though I somehow knew its spelling. On the other hand, although I could clearly see the book, I could not recall if anything had been written on its cover. I remembered it was red and there was a sense that it was an ancient text.

That morning, I searched the Internet for red books and ancient texts to see if something would spark my memory. I did come across *The Red Book*, the unpublished work of Swiss psychologist Carl Jung that was compiled mainly between 1914 and 1915. The year 1914 caught my attention because of another book I owned from that year, *The Impersonal Life* by Joseph Benner. The year 1914 had recently been showing up for me: on a magazine cover at the grocery store, on the license plate of a car, and on a decorative pillow in a friend's home. Jung is also the one who coined the term *synchronicity*.

A search of the word *giok* revealed it to be an Indonesian word meaning "jade." Jade is also the name we had chosen for our daughter, who is now in eternal sleep. Why would my subconscious mind give me a word that proved meaningful to me but in a foreign language, and at this time, 13 years after losing our daughter? I have never been to Indonesia, nor do I have any recollection of hearing that word before. Yet somehow it had emerged from the deeper parts of me. I also realize that had my dream figure simply said, "I give you Jade," I may not have given the symbol of the book much thought. Soon after, I discovered that the gemstone jade symbolizes a connection between the realms of heaven and earth. It was only through reviewing my journaled memories and exploring the key themes that I was able to discern the deeper meaning of the dream itself: that my Jade continues to be with me in spirit.

GUIDEPOSTS FOR DREAM RECALL AND JOURNALING

Guideposts are essential to beginning and developing any practice, particularly one with the purpose of healing and living our lives more fully. They empower us by requiring us to take regular action. For a dream journaling practice, there are four simple guideposts: awareness, compassion, trust, sharing.

Guidepost 1: Awareness

What we think about, we also dream about. Energy flows in the direction of wherever we place our awareness. One of my clients, a woman in her late 40s named Terra, said that she had very little dream recall. Within a week of our conversation, she started having vivid dreams that she was able to remember. She was curious and began recording her dreams. When we began our work together, she did not think she'd ever be able to remember her dreams, but us speaking regularly about dreaming, and her recording of dreams, led to her improving her dream recall. The decision to keep a dream journal shows that you are available and ready to pay attention to the messages of your inner consciousness.

Becoming more aware of your dreams will also inspire greater dream recall. Another client, Ty, said that he was unsure whether he had any dreams. When I assured him that we all dream, he shrugged. After multiple conversations, he shared that he was remembering one or two dreams each morning, though he noted that they made "little to no sense." It is key to recognize that dreams are not produced by the logical mind. The prefrontal cortex, the part of the brain responsible for logical reasoning, is less active when we sleep. We all have seemingly nonsensical dreams that function to make us aware that we are at least paying attention to our dreams. The more we pay attention, the more we begin to see emerging patterns and themes.

Guidepost 2: Compassion

Cultivating a lens of compassion allows us to explore our inner life with openness and curiosity. Even seemingly "bizarre" dreams that cause heightened emotional responses likely have something relevant to reveal to us. Nightmarish images that terrify us shed light on fear and anxiety or bring our attention to something we might be avoiding while we are awake. At times it is not that the dream image itself is scary, but rather the superstitions we associate with it, or even our personal history with that symbol.

Kinley, a first-year nursing student, dreamed of a boa constrictor. She was fearful, as she interpreted it as a bad sign. To her, snakes represented someone who could not be trusted. Consider the expression "He's a snake." Was her deeper wisdom cautioning her about someone in her life? And why a boa constrictor? Snakes are also relevant to health and medicine. This was her first year in nursing school. In Amerindian and Asian cultures, snakes represent renewal and the ability to transform challenges into opportunities. Kinley related this dream to her reservations about a budding relationship. While there was no obvious reason to distrust the man she was seeing, she was already feeling a sense of being smothered by his constant presence, leaving hardly any time to just chill with friends. A compassionate approach to our dreams allows us to recognize our immediate needs and what we value most. Instead of labeling a dream as "good" or "bad," the practice of self-compassion encourages our inner world to continually inform our waking lives.

Guidepost 3: Trust

Some dreams unfold over time. It requires a sense of trust to accept not knowing the immediate interpretation of a dream and to instead embrace the mystery of its unraveling. It could take weeks, months, or even years, as in the case of my dream of a fish inside a crib. Keeping a dream journal allows you to revisit the dream at a later time. I have often picked up an old journal and reread an entry only to uncover a new message or theme. Psychologist and dream expert Stephen Aizenstat, Ph.D., offers the idea of *dream tending*, where you encourage a specific dream image to continue to communicate its message while you are awake. It is the same as tending to a garden: We need to nurture it. Then we allow it to simply be, trusting nature to do what it does best, to draw forth life.

Guidepost 4: Sharing

The act of sharing your dream allows for further dream recall and insight. Even if you cannot remember much of your dream, details can come flooding back once you begin retelling it. In sharing your dreams with others, you give them the opportunity to consider what your dream might mean to them. They also get to witness and participate in the unfolding of your dream. For instance, once in a lucid dream I encountered a stranger who told me his name, which was an uncommon one in this day and age, but a popular one in the 1880s. Three days later, I actually encountered someone with this name. I had already shared about the dream with a few trusted friends. Each of them also came across the name: as a surname, as a woman's first name, and as a character in a mystery novel. A comment by another friend sparked this insight: What if it is less about the name but more about how abundantly thoughts manifest when others reveal their own thoughts?

Remember these four guideposts—awareness, compassion, trust, and sharing—when you are beginning your journey of inner exploration. Everyone dreams, and you do have the ability to remember. You do have the ability to learn and heal from what you discover. Like everything else, it requires practice.

WHEN TO RECORD YOUR DREAMS

Soon after waking is typically the best time to record the details, even if you do not have time to reflect on the message or symbolism. This is when you are closest to the dream, to the emotions, the felt sensations in your body, the phrases and words that presented themselves. This is when dream images are most intact. Though you might lose the details, the essence of the dream likely remains, and that is often enough for you to reflect upon. Take notice of your mood. Are you feeling peaceful and content? Are you feeling a bit unsettled or irritable? The most helpful thing to do is to sit with that vague awareness and a pen and paper, and write whatever streams into your consciousness.

There are times when we awaken in the middle of the night, and getting out of bed to write down a dream might interfere with our ability to fall back to sleep. Instead of leaving your bed, take a moment to review the dream, then focus your awareness on one particular image or person from the dream and make some association before going back to sleep. For example, if you dream of someone, think about the last time you saw that person. If you dream of being at the ocean, think back to the last time you were at the beach. There is a greater likelihood that your memory of that one image or person will be triggered by something throughout the day. Then, as soon as you're able to, sit down with your journal. Write what you remember, and more details may appear. A recent example of this is when I dreamed of driving alone in my car and coming from the other direction in her car was a friend I had not seen in months. I had forgotten this dream when I woke up and just went about my day. However, while checking my e-mails that morning, as soon as I saw my friend's name, I immediately recalled the dream.

What if you do not have time to record your dreams every morning? First of all, even if you are unable to recall the dream, know that it has served its purpose. If not, it will come again. Secondly, dream journaling does not require analysis. You are simply keeping a record. You can be as brief or as detailed as you wish. Coming up with a title that expresses the theme of a dream will also help to serve as future reference.

TIPS FOR STARTING YOUR DREAM JOURNALING PRACTICE

There is no one correct way to keep a dream journal. Practically speaking, find a journal that you like and adopt a format that works best for you. A downloadable dream journal is available on my website, kathleenomalleymessages.com, so you can begin right away. Keep in mind that even someone who ordinarily has great dream recall can experience periods of not remembering dreams. Unless dreams are being suppressed by medications or alcohol, you still experience the benefits of REM-sleep dreaming—consolidating memory, building connections, processing strong emotions, and solving problems, whether or not you can recall what you dreamed.

Keep your journal, a night-light, and a reliable writing pen next to your bed for easy access. Alternatively, you might choose to dictate your dreams into a recording device. Here are six simple steps to get started.

1. Set an intention

We will discuss the practice of dream incubation and asking for guidance in the next chapter. For now, here are a few examples: "I intend to have a restful night's sleep and wake up feeling ready to embrace a new day." "I intend to have greater clarity regarding . . ." I would appreciate any insight about . . ." "I would enjoy a visit from . . ."

2. Mentally commit to remembering your dreams

Simply state out loud as many times as you desire: "I will remember my dreams when I wake up." The repetition cements your intention, thereby increasing the chance of your wish becoming reality. It is that simple.

3. Tune in to your body as you awaken

Your body remembers what your mind quickly forgets. As you awaken, the key is to remain relaxed and still while becoming fully aware of your bodily sensations, the emotions you experienced, and replay as many details of your nightly vision as you can before getting up. Note that alarms and jarring sounds can impact dream recall. Try to establish a schedule so that you can awaken naturally. Prepare yourself for a good night's rest by avoiding electronics before bed, dimming the lights in preparation for bed, and going to sleep early.

4. Record the dream

There are numerous approaches when it comes to recording your dreams. You can highlight specific emotions and images that grab your attention: feelings, emotions, people, places, things, colors, symbols, numbers, spoken words, remnants of phrases, etc. Put pen to paper and don't worry if all the details come out in order. You could also record the dream as though you were sharing it with someone else, writing or speaking in the present tense. For example, *I am alone, walking alongside a quiet road, when I notice a cavernous pit . . .* or *I see myself standing inside my childhood home . . .* Write it all down—the setting, the timing, the people present, the conversations, the scents—without judging or attempting to analyze it. If your time is limited, simply write one or two images, anything that stood out that could prompt further recall of more details later. And if you are a visual person, consider drawing out your dream.

5. Create a title by identifying a theme

After recording what you remember, consider what the theme might be and create a title. The process of narrowing in on a theme or creating a dream title can be key to determining your dream's overall message. It can alert you to what patterns you might need to change or what action steps might be necessary at this time. Do not overthink it. Read what you wrote and let the message arise from within. It could be similar to a news headline: "Young Girl Encounters Crib with a Fish Inside." It could be a single word or even a phrase such as "Permission Granted" or "The Book of Jade." The more you practice this, the more intuitive this process becomes. Coming up with a title will also help you to return to the dream, particularly if something happens in your life that mimics the dream or if you have a similar dream in the future.

6. Notice synchronicities in your waking life

This is an important step, as it requires a greater awareness in your waking life. Take notice of any signs and synchronicities that show up throughout your day. This will allow you to connect your dreaming world with your waking world. I had a dream on May 28, 2020, of being on an archaeological expedition of some sort. It felt as though

I was in a foreign country. Later that day while writing, I referenced a quote a friend had once shared, "Not all the tree's blossoms will bear fruit." I researched the quote and learned that it was a Mauritanian proverb. When I looked up Mauritania, a country in northwest Africa, its sandy landscape reminded me of my dream setting. A synchronicity appeared two days later, when a clue in the Sunday crossword puzzle of our local newspaper read "Mauritania neighbor." Finding this clue felt as though the dream was still reaching out to me, causing me to return to that journal entry once more. I had titled the dream "Permission Granted," since I had received permission to obtain a sample of a valuable artifact on my dream expedition. However, I could not recall the artifact, leading me to believe that the dream was emphasizing the value of the exploration, the journey, the adventure, rather than a specific find or result. Not all blossoms may bear fruit, as the Mauritanian proverb suggests; still, they all deserve the chance to at least blossom.

Starting a dream journal can be daunting. This is the format I tend to use when recording my dreams. Try this, then mold it to serve your purposes and style.

Date: June 18, 2006
Day of Week: Sunday
Time: 5:55 a.m.

TITLE OF DREAM/THEME: *Mama's Message at the River's Edge*

PEOPLE/PLACES/THINGS: *Mama, a storm, on a cliff at the river*

FEELINGS/EMOTIONS: *(During or after waking) Cold and afraid*

COLORS: *The dark navy of night*

SYMBOLS: *Storm, scary cliff, wind, river*

DETAILS: *It is dark and stormy, and I am alone on a cliff. The winds are howling and strong. I am about to fall off the cliff when I hear Mama calling my name. I hear myself say yes as I wake up.*

INSPIRED ACTION STEPS/CHANGES/DECISIONS: *I am not alone, even in times when I feel most alone. The strength to face each day comes in knowing that I do not have to face grief and other challenges on my own.*

DREAM VISUALIZATION PRACTICE: REMEMBERING YOUR DREAM

Dreamscape: The following visualization practice, specific to dream recall, can be done either before bed or upon waking.

Objective(s): To practice body awareness and open your senses to the present moment in order to enhance your ability to remember your dreams

Visualization: Sit comfortably with your chest slightly lifted, allowing your shoulders to gently open and relax downward. Feel any tension in your shoulders slowly release. You might want to position your palms facing upward on your lap or on your knees, helping you to maintain this open posture.

See this body position as a way to open your heart to something bigger than yourself, the force of life that allows us all to exist as we are, a sense of community and shared purpose, a connection to a greater power.

Breathe deeply, receiving this nourishing breath in through the heart with every inhale. On the exhale, see this breath being released out through the heart.

Breathe in through the heart, deep into the belly, and breathe out through the heart.

Now as you breathe, visualize this nourishing, vitalizing breath flowing freely throughout the body, energizing every organ, every muscle, every cell in your body, before being released through the heart.

Continue breathing. Find a rhythm that is most comfortable for you.

Now we'll begin our visualization. Imagine yourself lying on a soft blanket in an open field, observing the moon-lit sky. Feel the texture of the blanket as you lie there, perhaps with your feet crossed at the ankles, your head resting on a comfortable pillow. You are held and supported by the earth. Feel its warmth. Know that you are completely safe. You are protected.

As you feel your body relaxing, tune in to the sounds of the night. What do you hear?

Do you hear the crickets singing in the distance? Or the sound of frogs in a nearby pond, or the call of a night owl?

Look up at the night sky and see the stars begin to appear. Some are just specks of light. Others are bright and luminous. What else do you see among the stars? Is your mind connecting them, making images?

Perhaps you see a shooting star or two or three. What do you wish for? Whisper that wish, knowing that it is heard only by the moon and the stars.

Now imagine falling asleep under this glorious starry sky. You begin to dream, and in your dream, you receive a visitor. Who is this person or being? Is this someone you know or have known? Is it a divine being or an ancestor? Is it someone at a distance you might be wanting to connect with?

Take a moment now and notice where you are. Are you still in the open field with this visitor or have you traveled? Are you somewhere else?

Take stock of how you feel in the moment. What sensations do you feel in your body in this person's presence?

What message does this person have for you?

Finally, know that your time here has come to an end. How do you say good-bye to this person?

Embodiment: Slowly bring your awareness back to your breath. Breathe in, breathe out, breathe in and out. Feel your feet on the floor, and slowly stretch your legs and your arms. Gently open your eyes or raise your gaze, returning to the present time and space, fully reinhabiting your body. Take note of how you feel in body, in mind, in heart.

I invite you to take a few moments to record the details of this experience: images, sounds, scents, bodily sensations, details about your conversation, and anything else you wish to remember about your exchange with this visitor. If you had to give this dream experience a title, what would the title be? Take as much time as needed to complete this process.

Chapter 2

DREAM INCUBATION AND ASKING FOR GUIDANCE

It was during the summer of 2009 when I learned we were expecting again. There were two dreams that caused me to suspect this pregnancy. In one dream, I was looking out my bedroom window, observing an unknown fisherman, when a runaway fish escaped his bucket and began to slide headfirst down our driveway. It was quite comical, and I woke up laughing. Next, I dreamed that my husband and I were at a stadium where a woman who had given birth to sextuplets was randomly selecting couples from the crowd to receive one of her newborn babies. We were the third couple chosen as parents to an infant boy.

With this pregnancy, I adopted a wait-and-see mindset—that is, waiting to share the news with family and friends. In previous pregnancies, I had sought early prenatal care, followed the recommendation for progesterone injections, ultrasounds, and other evaluations, yet the outcome was the same. In my sixth pregnancy, I was evaluated at 11 weeks gestation to see if an incompetent cervix was the reason for my recurring losses and was told it was not. I miscarried that pregnancy at 13 weeks. This time, I received prenatal acupuncture and other care, but felt trepidation about seeking obstetrical care. I considered reaching out to the midwife who had seen me through my only successful pregnancy, but I waited. I waited until 14 weeks into this pregnancy before asking my dreams for guidance. After journaling one night, I said a prayer and simply stated before I went to bed, "I need to know what to do. Show me."

Days later, in an early-morning dream, a male physician said to me, "You will not survive this pregnancy without having surgery." Though his demeanor was pleasant and calm, the declaration was startling and woke me right up. While I knew a hospital delivery would be advised given my extensive history and preterm deliveries, there was no apparent reason not to see my midwife for early prenatal care. However, soon after this dream, I experienced bleeding, which caused me to seek out the obstetrician who had evaluated me once before, Dr. D. She began following my pregnancy at about 16 weeks gestation. She advised progesterone injections and strict bed rest because of the unexplained bleeding. This is also when we learned we were expecting a son. I immediately thought of the dream of the fish sliding headfirst down our driveway. I imagined that one day I would watch our son go sledding down our driveway and caution him not to go headfirst.

At 21 weeks gestation, I was admitted to the hospital with premature ruptured membranes and told that labor was imminent. I was advised that the safest option for me would be to have my labor induced. This was right after hearing our son's heartbeat and being told that it was strong and that his movement was good. Just as in my dream of the sextuplets in the stadium, I believed I was chosen to be his mother. "It is possible for the membranes to seal," one nurse had said. "Miracles do happen," she offered. If there was any possibility of his survival, I needed to give him that chance, so I waited for labor to proceed without intervention. I waited, to allow him the time he needed to be of this world. I also needed this time with him.

INCUBATING

In biology, the term *incubation* is used to describe the period of time as well as the environment required to allow a process to reach full maturity. Birds incubate their eggs until they are ready to be hatched. Babies born before 37 weeks gestation are often placed in an incubator to allow for continued development of their lungs and other vital organs. Similarly, when you say, "Let me sleep on it," you are allowing your deeper consciousness the space to incubate a decision that aligns with your highest well-being. You can also be intentional by asking for specific guidance before or as you fall asleep.

The practice of dream incubation originated in ancient Greece. Travelers with health concerns would arrive at healing sanctuaries known as Asclepions. These sacred spaces were situated amid majestic gardens with elaborate fountains, mineral springs, theaters, and stadiums. After rituals that included nourishing foods, cleansing baths, exercises, and prayers, a person would go to sleep in a dream incubation chamber. While they slept, they would be visited by either Asclepius, the divine physician himself, or one of his totem animals, most often a snake or a dog. Dreamers might spend one day or multiple days at the Asclepion, returning to their dream chamber in the evenings. According to the inscriptions on the walls of these sanctuaries, dreamers would leave either fully healed or with specific instructions that led to their healing.

THE PATH TO HEALING

Imagine being in a serene, nurturing environment where you are well-nourished, undergo detoxification, given specific exercises, recite prayers or affirmations, and are allowed to sleep restfully. Any combination of these modalities could activate the body's innate healing response. A program designed to nourish, cleanse, strengthen, and give the body space to rest peacefully would do wonders for many of us. It is important to note that healing occurs not only with a specific cure but also when there has been a release of something that has blocked the body's natural restorative abilities. This includes past traumas, phobias, negative emotions or patterns, boundary issues, or other programming. When these overwhelming energies are released from the recesses of our inner world, our bodies can undergo much-needed repair and function more optimally.

One of my patients, a 32-year-old woman, was diagnosed with unexplained secondary infertility after a history of preterm labor and birth loss. She had already tried functional nutrition, herbs, and acupuncture, which had been helpful to her once before. I explained that there were no guarantees, but I would use every tool I had to help restore balance within her body. She consented to care and in addition to chiropractic adjustments, we used an approach known as Healing from the Body Level Up

(HBLU) to transform limiting beliefs and unwanted patterns. About six weeks later, she sent me this e-mail.

> Hi Dr. Kathy,
>
> I can't help but feel like you somehow knew last week that I am pregnant!
>
> I am a mix of thoughts, feelings, and emotions, but am so, so grateful for your guidance and support. Consider me a success story. . . . I'm not sure what it was that ultimately led to me finally being able to get pregnant, but I'm sure you had something to do with it.
>
> Thank you so much!
>
> Best,
> Annalee

Rarely is it ever just one thing that brings us to a state of well-being. Healing is an ongoing process that begins when we become aware of the deepest parts of ourselves that require our attention, when we are nourished and replenished and seek to transform our painful experiences. Healing occurs when we identify, fully acknowledge, process, and release anything that conceals our fullest expression. Healing is multidimensional, taking place in our physical body, our emotional body, our conscious and subconscious mind, and in ethereal and invisible dimensions. Healing happens when we are nurtured and fully supported without judgment or criticism. My patient is now the mother of four: one heavenly angel and three surviving children, two of them conceived after her diagnosis of secondary infertility.

As you contemplate asking your dreams for guidance, realize that healing may not come as neatly packaged as we might expect or exactly as we desire. There are times when life asks us to grow beyond current ways of thinking and existing. We are invited to remain curious, hopeful, and open to possibilities yet to be considered. In certain instances, it can feel less like an invitation and more of a reckoning, but when we can trust the process, we can participate in how it unfolds. "Miracles happen," told to me by a kind nurse, were the words I needed to hear in that stressful moment and provided much-needed calm and comfort. There is no such thing as false hope if it gets us through dark times and to a place of greater solidity. Hope reminds us to breathe and continue *lifeward,* toward that which sustains life. "My hope is that above all else, you continue to trust in the wisdom of your own body," was one of my responses to my patient's e-mail. If you are reading this, that is also my message to you. Trust in the wisdom of your body.

LETTING GO OF CERTAINTY

The incubation process also requires letting go of certainty and accepting the sensation of uncertainty. We are conditioned to reason and seek answers as a means of security. However, we live in an interconnected and constantly evolving universe. Sometimes there is no single answer, and often the answers are not what we expect. We truly have no other choice but to embrace the mystery. It doesn't have to be scary. Mysteries are a gift. Consider dreams: Even in the world of neuroscience, where advances in dream research are being made, dreams themselves remain a fascinating enigma. This mysterious nature of dreams allows each person to have singular experiences that are unique to them.

AN EXPERIENCE OF UNCONDITIONAL LOVE

The dream of being told I would not survive my current pregnancy without surgery was alarming, but I did not give it much attention at the time. Instead, I saw it as a directive that a high-risk obstetrician might be the best provider for me. My labor did progress on New Year's Day in 2010. After the birth of our son, who was stillborn, a post-delivery complication known as disseminated intravascular coagulation required me to have surgical interventions, blood and plasma transfusions, as well as intubation. The need to be ventilated was due to the fact that I had lost more than half of my blood volume, and inadequate blood flow meant inadequate oxygen levels. It was not until long after my recovery that I thought about the premonitory nature of that dream. Somehow my body knew that medical care would be required.

Holding another baby only to say good-bye was painful. Before that day, my prayer had been for him to be born healthy. As labor ensued, I spoke to him, saying that I would accept him however he came into this world, and that good health was not a condition for my love. It was soon after I expressed my unconditional love for him that the contractions began to intensify. I have often wondered if that is all he needed in this life, to be loved unconditionally.

He never took a breath and yet he breathed such meaning into my life. His essence typically comes to me in the form of recurring numbers. He was born on 1/1/10 at 11:10 P.M. Since then, whenever I notice 111 and 1110, there is a sense of being guided by a larger presence. When I shared his birth certificate on my blog, someone pointed out that the attending physician's registry number also ended in 111. It feels as though this is his way of reminding me that we are forever connected. He will always be my son and I will forever be his mother. Even if I knew beforehand the length of time we would have had together in this physical realm, I can now say with certainty that I would have still chosen to have had that time with him. It has taken much healing and growth to arrive at acceptance. Note that acceptance does not mean we can always be grateful for the experience. It means that we make peace with the fact that the experience unfolded in the way that it did. The other message that comes with acceptance—and then healing—is that even when we get a glimpse of what the future might hold, we still must take the necessary steps to get there.

ASKING FOR GUIDANCE

Asking your dreams for guidance expresses trust in your body's internal navigation system and trust in the unseen presence that brought us all into being. Dream incubation begins with formulating a specific question, a prayerful intention or thought you wish to explore more deeply in your dream world. Then you focus on that intention, either silently or aloud, as you fall asleep. Your intentions can incubate specific dreams in the same way that your daily activities and experiences can influence your nightly visions. You might even choose to design your dreamscape by calling to mind a specific setting, familiar or imagined. You might request a specific visitor such as a loved one who has passed on, an ancestor, or a divine being. You can also simply just state your intention. Then you must let go of time lines, of expectations. Sometimes the guidance is immediate. Other times it takes days, weeks, or longer for the guidance to evolve and unfold. Trust that your dreams will know when and how to provide the best guidance and in the most suitable way imaginable.

Your inner wisdom is in constant communication with all parts of your being. It can easily sort through files of stored information to best integrate and provide meaningful insights. As you sleep, not only does your body naturally undergo healing processes, but your brain can also interpret subtle signals of dis-ease and then formulate images that are reflected in your dreams. This is your body's innate ability to protect and guide you toward healing. In his book *The Neuroscience of Sleep and Dreams,* Patrick McNamara, an associate professor of neurology at Boston University, explains how illnesses and other dysfunctions in the body can be revealed via one's thoughts or dreams even before they can be detected by conventional means. A seemingly random thought about a specific health concern, then, might warrant further investigation, even if you do not recall any dream images. Pay attention to any sensations you feel in your body when you awaken. This will help you develop the ability to attune to your body's wisdom and give credence to spontaneous messages that you receive.

LISTENING TO THE BODY'S MESSAGES

Symptoms are messengers. Any form of pain, tension, or discomfort is often the body's way of signaling your attention to an underlying imbalance. But we usually disregard any pain until it (hopefully) goes away or try to numb the discomfort in some way. This does not mean that you must suffer needlessly if there is a remedy or technique that can provide relief. It means that you *listen* to your bodily sensations. You allow yourself the comfort you need as you examine the underlying cause of your discomfort. That ache in your neck and shoulders might warrant a change in your posture, and it might be signaling to you that psychological burdens have become too heavy to carry on your own. That uneasiness you feel in your solar plexus might be a digestive issue, and it might be signaling your attention to unprocessed emotions that have been stuffed down over the years. Pain and discomfort could be a sign of overuse and a call to rest and restore, or a sign of deficiency, reminding you to nourish and replenish.

While your dreams can often initiate awareness, it is up to you to heed these calls and take appropriate action. The sensations in your body can help you understand underlying needs, your ways of functioning, as well as your deepest motivations. As such, take note of any sensations that are with you when you awaken, the ones that remain with you throughout the day, and any that surface. Where is each sensation located in the body? Assign a number to the intensity of each sensation, rating them on a scale of 1 to 10, with 10 being the most intense. What feelings or emotions arise as you continue to focus your awareness? Allow each sensation to lead and guide you by paying attention to the thoughts that spontaneously enter your mind when you are focused on a particular sensation. I encourage you to make notes throughout your day, and when you have time, engage in deeper reflection. You can continue this exploration through writing or in sharing with a trusted loved one. Or consider consulting a professional. Keep in mind that self-compassion is a requirement as you explore the messages that you receive. Also, practice patience as you allow these messages to unfold and reveal themselves to you.

STEPS FOR INCUBATING YOUR DREAMS

There are four steps to incubating dreams for guidance and healing.

1. Write
2. Recite
3. Record
4. Replay

Write

The process of writing invites whatever is unexpressed to the surface in order for you to better understand the world within you. Begin by sitting in silence. Then write the mix of emotions that you are experiencing, as well as any thoughts that stream into your consciousness. As you write, take notice of the sensations in your body and the shifts that occur as you continue this process. Next, read aloud what you have written. This provides even greater clarity as it engages even more of your senses. Sound provides vibration, which enables us to feel whether or not something resonates.

Consider everything you have written to determine one specific area of your life that requires guidance or some form of healing. Finally, write down a focused intention in your dream journal before going to bed.

Recite

Recite your intention to receive guidance as you fall asleep. Because the subconscious mind is wide awake and listening as your conscious mind drifts to sleep, reciting an affirmation or intention right before sleep is empowering. This can be done silently or aloud. You might also play a recording through earphones of a dream you wish to incubate that includes specific details of your dream setting, as well as the dream figures you wish to communicate with.

Record

When you awaken in the morning, remain as still as possible as you recall the details of your dream. Take note of any sensations in your body. Record your feelings, images that you remember, words or phrases that were offered to you in your dream, anything at all. If it resonates, assign a title to the dream. Finally, record any synchronicities that show up in your waking life. Did someone mention something that reminded you of your dream? How often did one of the images from your dream continue to show up over the course of a week?

Replay

Keep the same intention night after night until you receive clear guidance. If something else becomes more of a priority, feel free to create a new intention and allow this new intention to replay until guidance is received.

The more you engage with your dreams, the more you will discover the interconnected nature of our existence. Keep in mind that you dream about five to eight dreams each night. Even the ones you do not recall can hold indeterminate benefits.

Remember the guideposts for dream recall: awareness, compassion, trust, sharing. Wherever you place your awareness, energy will flow. Have compassion for yourself as you evolve and grow in understanding of your dreams. Trust that the guidance will come not always as you expect but in the best way possible. Share with others not only to hear their insights but also to hear yourself more clearly.

CREATING YOUR DREAMSCAPE

I invite you to take some time now to consider a dream you would like to incubate. First, what is your intention? Is there a specific question you would like to ask your deeper self while you sleep? Is there a health concern that you would like to receive guidance about? Is there a situation that has been troubling to you or to someone you love? Is there someone you would like to have a visit from in your dreams?

Take a few moments to record your intention:

_____

_____

_____

_____

_____

_____

DREAM VISUALIZATION PRACTICE: DREAM INCUBATION FOR GUIDANCE AND HEALING

Dreamscape: A healing sanctuary with sacred dream chambers, surrounded by gardens of blossoming fruit trees, flowers, and herbs, as well as a nearby spring with crystalline waters

Objective(s): To experience the practice of dream incubation that originated in ancient Greece, and to set clear intentions for guidance you wish to receive in your dream state

Visualization: Sit comfortably, allowing your shoulders to gently open, with your chest slightly lifted. You might position your palms facing upward on your lap or on your knees to help you maintain this open posture.

Gently close your eyes or lower your gaze and bring your awareness to your heart.

With every inhale, imagine your breath entering through the heart, traveling deep into the belly. With every exhale, see your breath being released through the heart.

Breathe in, through the heart, deep into the belly, and out through the heart. Receive this nourishing, vitalizing breath into the heart.

Whatever thoughts arise, allow them to float in and out. Gently draw your attention back to the breath.

Breathe deeply, allowing this breath to transfuse every system in your body—every organ, every tissue, every cell.

Continue breathing, finding a rhythm that is most comfortable for you.

Imagine that you have just arrived at a healing sanctuary surrounded by a tranquil garden of blossoming fruit trees, shrubs, herbs, and flowers of every color.

Breathe deeply, inhaling the scent of lavender or other aroma that is soothing to your senses.

Hear the soft sound of flowing water from a nearby stream.

Turn to look to the horizon, noticing the sky turning from orange and red to a lilac afterglow as day fades into night.

Take a deep breath of the cool night air before ascending a flight of granite stairs. At the top of the stairs, you are greeted and invited into the sanctuary.

You are led to a private room that has been prepared for you to experience a ritual cleansing bath. There is a copper tub filled with crystalline water from a nearby spring with added salts, herbs, flower essences, and petals. There is also a footbath where you can sit comfortably and soak your feet.

You get to decide how much of yourself you would like to submerge in these healing waters. Whichever you choose, allow these waters to soothe and comfort you, helping you to release all that is beyond your control, all that no longer serves your highest expression.

Be softened by these healing waters, allowing yourself to become as fluid and as flexible as this water, feeling every muscle in your body, from the tops of your shoulders to the tips of your toes; relax and let go. Imagine the worries of the day dissolving as easily as the bath salts did. Feel a sense of ease, of releasing, of cleansing, of allowing.

Whenever you are ready to emerge from your bath, see yourself prepared for sleep, wearing comfortable sleepwear.

Imagine being led to your own chamber, a private room with a bed and a rocking chair with a blanket. Notice the corner table with a single lit candle and a cup of your favorite tea.

Sit for a while, sipping on your tea if you choose. Take a few moments to consider what guidance and healing insights you would like to receive while you sleep.

Now see yourself rising from the chair and getting into the cozy bed. It molds to your body and seems as though it was made just for you.

Now imagine falling asleep in your dream chamber. What guidance and healing insights do you receive?

Embodiment: When you are ready, imagine yourself slowly beginning to wake up in your dream chamber. Feel yourself becoming more aware. Gently open your eyes and remain still for just a while longer. Now slowly move and stretch your body, your arms, your legs. See yourself fully awake, feeling renewed and rested.

Fully reinhabit this present time and space, stretch your body, and take note of bodily sensations and emotions. I encourage you to record your experience of this practice. What guidance and healing insights did you receive? In what form were these messages delivered? Who or what was the messenger?

Chapter 3

UNDERSTANDING THE MESSAGES YOU RECEIVE

February 1, 2010: *I am in an unfamiliar room, and I find myself waiting. It is not clear who or what I am waiting for. I hear a gentle tapping at the door. I approach the door only to stand before it in silence. My pulse quickens as I wait. I make no attempt to answer the knock until a whispered voice says, "It is me." This is when I open the door.*

This dream was clearly a metaphor for all that was happening. A childhood friend had offered to be a gestational surrogate for me and my husband. We met when she was eight and I was nine. We lived across the street from each other on the island of Saint Thomas, attended the same schools, and shared a similar background. Our mothers knew each other. Our grandmothers knew each other. Aside from my grandmother, she is the only other person with whom I had consistently shared my nighttime dreams, particularly in middle school, when my dreams were mostly fantastical. It became our ritual. Her dad would drive us to school early, I would tell her my dreams, and most often she would fall to the floor, laughing. We kept in touch through college and after. We visited each other after our daughters were born, 15 months apart. Yet my initial reaction to her offer was no. *That is not the way nature intended it,* was my initial thought. "A child should be created out of love," I had said in response to her offer.

With time, my perspective did shift as I recognized that this truly was an act of love. A trusted friend was willing to help me in bringing a desired child into the world. Why would I not accept this beautiful gift? It was easier for my husband to come to this decision than it was for me. I had to replace a long-held dream—the natural childbirth experience I had once imagined. I had to open to other views of conception and see assisted reproduction as a miraculous process. This would also be the ultimate lesson in letting go. So much would be beyond my control.

WHAT IF THIS WERE YOUR DREAM?

When it comes to understanding the messages of your dreams, recognize that you hold the key to fully connecting the imagery and the emotions experienced in a dream with your waking reality and your creative potential. Dreams take everything you have ever known, your past experiences, your history, cultural background, beliefs, values, as well as our collective experience—all that is stored within us and beyond us. And then, as though directed by a creative muse, dreams weave together a series of connections that allow for brilliant solutions, artistic expressions, and unique landscapes.

Though we all have similar behaviors and patterns, no one has experienced life exactly as you have. Likewise, it is not up to you to interpret the meaning of someone else's dream. One way to begin exploring the wisdom of dreams is, whenever you hear or read about someone else's dream, ask yourself: What if this were my dream?

SYMBOLISM, MYTH, METAPHOR

Dreams allow us to express ourselves in the most creative ways. Our dreaming mind makes connections that clearly extend beyond the scope of our logical mind. Symbolism, myth, and metaphor add perspective, yet allow us to go beyond what is known. They encourage the dreamer to observe and remain curious rather than label dream imagery as either good or bad, negative or positive. In the introduction I shared the dream that communicated my daughter's conception, of a fish swimming in the sky. Why did this dream choose the sky and not the ocean to highlight the fish? Was it simply to capture my curiosity? Many of us have heard the phrase "a fish out of water" used as a negative connation to express vulnerability and uncertainty, yet this dream offered certainty and a positive correlation in my reality.

Often, we can relate aspects of a dream to occurrences in our waking lives. Other times it seems as though we are given pieces of a puzzle, only to find that the range of possibility is endless. Consider the symbol of a door. A closed door might represent a time of transition, often an ending, or it could indicate that something is not available to you. From the perspective of being on the inside, a firmly closed door might be offering you protection and security. That is, if you feel safe and protected in the dream, not trapped or claustrophobic. What about an open door?

In ancient Rome there is a deity known as Janus who typically symbolizes doorways, gates, and other passageways. Janus is often depicted as having two faces, indicating the possibility of a beginning or an ending, a transition to or from another stage. The doors of Janus's shrine were opened when the Roman army was at war and closed in times of peace. While you might think that doors should be closed during times of war to offer protection, the open shrine door was thought to allow peace to be sent outward to those engaged in war. During peaceful times, closing the shrine doors represented the desire to not yield to war but to keep imprisoned all that came with war.

There is also the adage that "When one door closes, another opens," to which Helen Keller adds, " . . . but often we look so long at the closed door that we do not see the one which has opened for us."[1] The key point is to recognize that dreaming is a dynamic force that encourages a wider perspective and deeper understanding in our waking lives. We look to adages for the wisdom of those who came before us. Still, we live in changing times and have our own experiences. For you in the here and now, a closed door may just mean that you have the option of choosing whether or not to unlock and open that door. What if an open door makes logical sense and yet the deepest part of you calls you elsewhere?

ALLOWING THE DREAM TO UNFOLD

Though a dream might offer a new perspective, inspire a particular action, or point you in a certain direction, try to not seek one specific interpretation. Rather, keep an open mind and allow the dream to evolve. Sometimes you are given just enough guidance to set you on a path that aligns with who you are in that moment, only to find that it goes in a completely different direction, one that you didn't expect—but that leads to even greater inner alignment.

In my case, the series of legal, psychological, and medical steps leading up to the surrogacy process seemed enormous. While my friend's one and only pregnancy had been uncomplicated, she still had to undergo thorough evaluations to determine if she was a good candidate for gestational surrogacy and that she would not be taking any undo risks "medically or emotionally." I felt overwhelming gratitude for her willingness to endure this process, even after learning about what it truly entailed. There were many reasons not to move forward with this complicated process. Yet there was an extraordinary sense of being divinely led in this specific direction.

After months of introspection, research, guidance, and prayer, it felt right to take this opportunity. "The odds are in your favor," the doctor had said. Each step leading up to the first attempt at surrogacy went better than expected. What once felt like a whispered yes seemed to resonate much louder. During this time, I also recalled the dream from years earlier of the woman who had given birth to sextuplets and chose my husband and me as parents for one of her infant sons. Was this the way it was supposed to finally happen? The timing felt right, and I was willing to endure the medical interventions and embrace this next chapter—though I still had some reservations.

At the time of our meeting to sign consent forms, I made it clear that I was willing to try this only once. *If this was meant to be, it should happen with the first attempt*, was my belief. We had already been through so much disappointment, and I could not imagine repeated treatment cycles. At first, I opposed the idea of any embryos being frozen for future use. My husband helped me see that it was reasonable just in case I felt differently later on. Reluctantly I agreed, but silently hoped that this would not be the case. Even when the ultrasound technician remarked, "Your ovaries are blossoming," prior to my egg retrieval, I prayed that there would be only one embryo.

On the morning of April 10, 2011, we received the call that a developing embryo was ready to be transferred. The best-case scenario would have been to transfer a single embryo, but no more than two. A single embryo had reached the blastocyst stage and was selected to be transferred. This embryo was placed into my friend's uterus by means of a catheter inserted through the cervix, guided by ultrasound. She reached out to hold my hand during the process. Everything went as planned. I was given an ultrasound printout and the date of our pregnancy test, April 22, 2011. For 11 nights, I hoped to dream of fish. Not only were there no fish dreams but I also struggled to remember the details of any of my dreams. I remained hopeful, feeling that this would be another lesson in patience.

INSIGHTS UPON WAKING

Even with no or suboptimal dream recall, bodily sensations, feelings, and spontaneous thoughts can still offer guidance. As discussed with dream incubation, the emotions and impressions present upon waking can assist you in uncovering images of your dreams and connect you to the messages you received. Is there a feeling of sadness or sense of contentment when you first open your eyes? Do you feel irritable for no apparent reason? Unsettled? Hopeful? What thoughts spontaneously enter your mind? Are you inspired to create? Do you find yourself humming a particular song? Are you thinking of someone you have not seen in a long while?

Though I could not recall the details of my dream on the morning of the embryo transfer, I had also awakened with thoughts of writing a book. This book would chronicle our experience of surrogacy. *My Baby, Her Body* was the title I wrote in my journal before heading to the fertility clinic. While that book did not materialize, I did follow through with my early-morning inspiration, which led to my first book—*Messages from Within: Finding Meaning in Your Life Experiences.*

The transition from sleep to waking is known as the hypnopompic state or hypnopompia. In the hypnopompic state, the brain attempts to search for known associations, even though the dreamer is unable to recall a specific dream. In this state, the whirring of a ceiling fan can bring to mind a helicopter, or a musical alarm might cause you to awaken with thoughts of being at a concert. However, an early-morning thought with no obvious association is likely dream-inspired. Some poets and songwriters awaken with lengthy stanzas or lyrics clear in their minds and ready to be written out but have no visual images or memory of a dream.

The morning of our pregnancy test, again I could not recall any dreams. This is likely because I had been so nervous, I barely slept that night. In my morning meditation, the image of a sand dollar came to mind. This seemed so out of the blue, I had to look up the symbolism. I learned that it was a lucky omen, and that it represented the birth, death, and resurrection of Christ. That day happened to be Good Friday, the Christian holiday that recognizes the crucifixion. Around 2 that Friday afternoon (April 22, 2011), a nurse telephoned with the result of the pregnancy test. It was negative.

CREATING YOUR OWN DREAM DICTIONARY

Now when I consider the message of the sand dollar, two things come to mind. The first is that some sand dollars must be returned to the ocean from which they came, for even after death the shell of a sand dollar benefits the ocean. The other is the legend of the doves of peace. This is when a nonliving sand dollar is cracked open to find five dove-shaped pieces that used to be the sand dollar's teeth. As the doves emerge, they are said to spread peace. For me, doves symbolize my grandmother's presence. To dream of a sand dollar might also reflect the connection I feel to her, reminding me that she is forever present to me. "I am the sea," she once offered to me in a dreamlike meditation.

When it comes to creating your own dream dictionary, start with symbols or images that are most meaningful to you. What image or images connect you to a loved one who is no longer present in this realm? What would a dream of a car or other vehicle mean to you? Do you find yourself dreaming of the ocean or other body of water when you have been feeling overwhelmed? Other than pregnancy, what might a dream of a baby indicate in your life?

Date: August 5, 2021
Day of Week: Thursday
Time: 4:38 a.m.

TITLE OF DREAM/THEME: *Retelling a First Dream within a Third Dream of the Night*

PEOPLE/PLACES/THINGS: *Baby, sofa chair, old friend, grapes, unknown woman, newspaper, current friend, the beach, church gathering*

FEELINGS/EMOTIONS: *(During or after waking) Joy and concern*

COLORS: *Green*

SYMBOLS: *Baby, grapes*

DETAILS: *In the first dream, I am on the beach and meet an old friend who has seven young children (in reality, she only has two). I offer to hold her infant boy. I am overcome with joy as I hold him close. There is a sofa chair at the beach. I place the baby on the sofa chair and leave him unattended. I return to see that he is holding a green grape in his hand. I then notice a gap in the back of the sofa chair with other grapes. I feel a sense of concern about what could have happened if he had placed the grape into his mouth.*

In a second dream, I'm walking in my neighborhood but stop at the side of a street to read a newspaper. An unknown woman is pushing a stroller along the same street. She stops to talk and says that she has enjoyed being a part of a writer's group during the pandemic that I might also enjoy. "How do you know I'm a writer?" I ask. "If you're a reader, you're a writer," she responds.

In a third dream, I am again at the beach. This time there is a church gathering (which has never occurred at a beach). I am leaving the event with a dear friend. As we walk, I proceed to tell her about the dream I had of the baby, the sofa chair, and the grapes.

INSPIRED ACTION STEPS/CHANGES/DECISIONS: *As I explore these dreams, I recognize that I would never leave a baby unattended on a sofa chair. However, I will often place my journal or a book on a sofa. I am currently working on this chapter, and as I write, there is a sense of being pregnant with knowledge and guidance. As for the grapes, I'm not sure. I have not eaten green grapes in a while, so I will allow this image to evolve.*

When I shared about this dream with a friend, she expressed that a baby in her dreams has often symbolized a creative pursuit. Had this been her dream, the overall message to her would have been, "All will be well." The baby did not fall from the sofa chair, nor did he place the grape into his mouth. If this had been her dream, she would have expected to encounter minor challenges with the knowing that everything would work out in the end.

Whenever an image in a dream, meditation, or spontaneous thought captures your interest, rather than seeking one obvious interpretation, remain open to other possibilities. Consider turning your attention to a dream character or an image that is less significant and see what guidance further emerges. Write down what comes to mind without worrying about what you are writing down. Look for any associations that can be made to your waking life and how you might apply the guidance received from a seemingly trivial dream image. Here is another example of this process:

January 13, 2021: *I'm in what appears to be a thrift store. I'm walking through racks of clothing that might have been worn by others. As I head toward the front of the store, I notice a round table. Its tablecloth print is of apples. My awareness moves from the table to three elderly women standing together at the front of the store. I make eye contact with one of the women. I do not recognize her face, but I seem to recognize her eyes.*

What captures my curiosity most is the eyes. The first thing that comes to mind is the saying, "Eyes are the windows to the soul." The next thought I have is the South African greeting of deep witnessing, *Sawubona,* which means "I see you. I respect you. I value you. You are important to me." One possible message: Though I made eye contact with just one, they all saw me. I am valued by all of the women in my lineage. I feel a warm sensation radiate through me with this interpretation.

The least significant image in this dream is the apples printed on the tablecloth. A quote attributed to Martin Luther King, Jr. is what I think of first. "Even if I knew that tomorrow the world would go to pieces, I would still plant my apple tree."[2] My next thought: You cannot fully predict or change tomorrow, but you can bring peace to this present moment and choose life.

This is how these symbols appear in my dream dictionary:

Apple: A reminder to be present, to choose life, to stay in integrity and reflect the peace I wish to see in the world; a symbol of deep commitment to inner peace

Eyes: A symbol of deep connection

THE IMPACT OF DAYTIME RESIDUE

The stories we hear and tell in our waking states often find their way into other states of consciousness, including our dreams. Had I read or watched any depiction of the fairy tale *Snow White* in the preceding days, my brain might have offered a much different presentation of the apple, a symbol that is central to that story but that appeared in my dream as a background image. Similarly, day-to-day concerns, unfinished tasks, conversations, and other interactions can also impact our dreaming landscape.

As discussed with dream incubation, pre-bedtime writing to take inventory and sort through emotions, thoughts, and bodily sensations, as well as to express gratitude can allow you to enter sleep with a greater sense of calm and inner peace. Even so, memories of the past and conversations from long ago can resurface in dreams. An incident that did not seem to be a big deal can be highlighted during our nighttime visions. How the dreaming mind ultimately links and blends everything together holds a lot of information for us.

The idea of sorting through our emotions and events of our day right before bed might seem counterintuitive to some. You might ask: Wouldn't this prevent me from getting to sleep? Actually, sometimes getting thoughts on paper can be the best way to calm the mind. It can be a difficult task to try not to think or worry about circumstances that impact our lives and the lives of our loved ones. Writing down our thoughts allows us to give them the recognition they need so that we can then put them aside to be addressed at a more appropriate time. What is truly amazing about this process is that oftentimes your dreams will do some of the work for you, even if you do not recall them.

THE VOICE OF YOUR INNER BEING

Now, more than 10 years later, when I reflect back to the voice at the door that said, "It is me," there is a sense of that voice being my own—the ever-evolving aspect of myself calling me onto a path the more familiar me might not have ordinarily taken. This deeper part of myself desires to experience all that this life has to offer regardless of outcomes; to replace "either/or" with "and." I did not initially recognize this voice as my own because I had yet to integrate that aspect of who I have become. With further growth and healing, this voice is now more easily recognizable. It is a voice from the depths of my being, yet it extends beyond me. It is the voice that allows me to guide others, not just as far as I have come, but rather it encourages me to lead them inward so that they might listen to and hear the callings of their own fertile being and carve their own path.

Your own inner being is constantly providing guidance. The challenge is distinguishing this voice from the beliefs, opinions, and expectations of others. While we do need other perspectives, you must be careful to never lose yourself. It does not serve anyone if you bury your own inner sense in response to what others say or do. That inner sense is what guides and liberates you from the conflicting messages that are outside of you. In your dream states, you are less encumbered by these outside voices. With your eyes closed, you are more open to your inner vision, your own intuition. You can see beyond current life circumstances and gather a wider perspective. You are able to hear what was previously inaudible. You are able to feel more deeply, to express a greater sense of aliveness as you experience the wonders of this life.

DREAMING WHILE AWAKE

Your inner wisdom does not only speak in nighttime dreams—it communicates through premonitions, whispers of intuition, and during meditative states. Whether in a sitting meditation, walking among the trees, or during a seemingly mindless task such as folding laundry, "The quieter you become," writes 13th-century Sufi mystic and poet Rumi, "the more you are able to hear."[3]

How will you recognize your innermost voice of inspiration and guiding wisdom? Listen and you will hear. This voice will not judge, criticize, or belittle you or anyone else. It gives and sustains life. It is not hurried, propelling you into irreversible action. It allows you to pause and wait for as long as necessary. It permits you to question rather than simply conform. It permits you to access and discover what is most essential to you in this moment.

"What did you and God talk about this morning?" my friend had asked. We were on our way back from the fertility clinic after the second embryo transfer. Yes, I had said I would do this procedure only once. However, between the time of the first embryo transfer and the first pregnancy test, I had received a letter from the fertility clinic. The letter informed us that two additional embryos had continued to grow on the day of the first transfer, and they were frozen for later use. My friend assured me that she would be willing to do this again. And we did.

The plan this time was to implant the remaining embryos. Again, the procedure went well, and I was given an ultrasound image but noticed there was only one cellular structure. I said to the nurse, "I assume the other embryo did not survive the thawing process." She looked at me questioningly. I explained further that there had been two embryos that were frozen, and we agreed to have both implanted this time. She left the room to consult with the doctor and returned to say that only one embryo had been thawed, and the doctor would contact me. He did. He explained that there had been a miscommunication, and this had never happened at his facility before. He seemed genuinely upset and assumed full responsibility, offering to cover the expense of a subsequent transfer, and wished me the best with our current pregnancy attempt.

To answer my friend's question about what God and I had talked about that morning: In prayer and meditation, I simply asked that God be present. This time I did not ask for a particular outcome. Here is what I had written in my journal the morning of the second transfer:

> June 13, 2011: *My thoughts today are focused on the transfer. We should get the call soon to say whether or not it will still happen (depending on whether the embryos survive the thawing process). What dwells in me at this time is a sense of hope. Faith and hope are all that I have when nothing else is for certain. I can't imagine that I was led down this road for no reason. It is my greatest desire to be a mother again. So, I trust that this is the way it is meant to happen. There is one other lesson that I am quite certain that I have learned. From this point on, I will be cautious about how I use the word* never. *I had said* never *to this entire process. I had said I would never want to do this again. Yet here I am. It seems that when I use that word, life gives me an opportunity to prove myself wrong.*

I no longer believe that life's intention is about proving us wrong. Rather, it is about expanding our imaginations, allowing ourselves to dream new dreams and continue to trust ourselves, others, the infinite intelligence of God, and the process of living this life. It is about opening less predictable doors in order to willingly participate in the extraordinary experiences that life often presents to us.

It was early in the afternoon on June 23, 2011, when the nurse called with the results of this pregnancy. I answered the phone in the kitchen. I was alone. I stood still. I caught myself holding my breath as I waited to hear the results after we exchanged greetings. My heart began to race. "We did get a positive," she said, "although the numbers were not as high as we would like to see them." She explained that she had seen numbers like these before that resulted in a live birth and continued to say that we should be "cautiously optimistic." The test would have to be repeated on the following Monday to see if the pregnancy hormone levels continued to rise.

Again, the results were not as we had hoped. The pregnancy was not progressing. During this call, the nurse also inquired about our intention to move forward with the final embryo transfer. When she said that I did not have to give an immediate answer, I was relieved. I did not have an answer. About a week later, I prayerfully asked for guidance not from my dreams but from my waking life—I wished for a sign. A few hours later, the guidance came in the form of a song by Kris Allen, "Live Like We're Dying." This song seemed to say not to let anything go undone. I could have interpreted this to mean that I should not delay moving forward. There had been so much disappointment that my usual tank of hope was depleted. When I thought of moving forward there was a feeling of defeat. It was as though an aspect of me was whispering, "Okay, let's just do it and get it over with." That was not the voice I wanted to listen to. I did not want to enter this amazing process with the energy of depletion. So I had my answer. It felt right to wait. And that is what we did.

GUIDELINES FOR ENGAGING WITH DREAMS

Our dreams are sacred because they come from an abundant source that exists within each of us, one that contains love, humor, and creativity. Give to your dreams the dignity that they deserve. As you seek to understand the messages you receive, let this be your oath.

1. **Observe** without judgment whatever your dream images bring to mind. Pay attention to when these images reappear in your waking life.

2. **Allow** for other possible interpretations. Permit the dream to evolve and unfold.

3. **Trust** in the wisdom of your inner being. It will guide you as far as you are ready to go.

4. **Honor** all aspects of yourself that show up in your dreams, even the parts that might terrify you.

DREAM VISUALIZATION PRACTICE: DOOR MEDITATION FOR MINDFUL DECISION-MAKING

Dreamscape: Standing before a closed door, you are guided to observe all the emotions and sensations associated with a decision you are currently facing. It could be a small decision or a major one. How might it feel if this door remained closed? And how might it feel to open the door?

Objective: To become attuned to your deepest wisdom and receive clear insight about a decision. To practice paying attention to your bodily sensations.

Visualization: Sit comfortably with your chest slightly lifted, shoulders relaxed, open palms, open heart, open mind.

I invite you to close your eyes and open to your inner vision.

Breathe deeply, finding a rhythm that works for you. Slowly bring your heart, your body, and your mind to a state of ease and calm.

See yourself standing before a door.

Notice the texture of the door, its color, the door handle or knob.

Continue to breathe in and out . . .

Allow any sensations or thoughts to arise spontaneously.

What sensations do you feel in your body as you stand before this door? Do you feel warmth or coolness in your body? Do you feel unsettled or comfortable?

Allow yourself to think about what might be on the other side of the door. What awaits you? It could be the answer to your question, a solution to your decision, a long-held dream.

Continue to consider what it might feel like if this door remained closed, if the mystery remained hidden.

Listen deeply. Listen with all your senses, with your whole being. Hear your innermost voice, your deepest wisdom, and the divine wisdom that transcends yet connects each of us.

What would it feel like to open this door?

What sensations arise? How do you feel in your body?

Finally, what wisdom do you hear? What are you being guided to do?

Embodiment: When you are ready, return to this present time and space. Move and stretch your body. Then, take as much time as you need to write about your experience of this practice, and consider whether you are closer to making a decision.

I encourage you to set the intention for more insight while you sleep. Return to this practice as needed.

Chapter 4

WHY WE HIDE, RUN, FALL, AND FLY

Rumi's quote "The quieter you become, the more you are able to hear" echoes once more. On the edges of sleep is often when we can hear most easily. In the stillness of the morning, I heard a whispered breath say, "I'm sorry—tell your mother." This immediately woke me up. My heart was racing, but there were no images or other context, just this apparent apology. Thoughts of my biological father began entering my mind. I knew only a few details about him: his name, the country he originated from, and that he had been deported from the country of my birth. I was 12 years old when I learned of him but did not ask any questions at the time. Instead, my preadolescent mind imagined that I was a product of young lovers who could not raise their baby together simply because they were from two different countries. The stories we tell are those we come to believe.

Now, decades later, it seemed my dreaming mind was attempting to tell a different story. This dream prompted me to ask questions about my parentage for the first time ever. At the age of 35, I learned that my mom had conceived as a result of having been violated. She was just 17. He was a much older man, a friend of the family. My mom was able to hide her pregnancy until just weeks before I was born. I couldn't help but wonder if this was why I was prone to dreams of hiding. As psychiatrist R.D. Laing writes in his book *The Facts of Life*, "The environment is registered from the very beginning of my life; by the first one (cell) of me."[1]

HIDING IN DREAMS

We hide when we are afraid. We hide when we feel ashamed of our identity, our missteps, our deficiencies, our apparent flaws, our apparent failures, our unrealized dreams. We hide because at our core we need to feel safe and secure. We hide to escape being ridiculed or reprimanded for not measuring up, for not getting it right, for not fitting into the acceptable mold. We also hide to preserve our sense of self, to protect our vulnerabilities from criticism and hurt. Even as we hide, there is a hope that the "danger" will pass or that we will be found and rescued. Or maybe we'll have the strength to devise a plan to rescue ourselves and no longer require protection. No matter what, we hide even though we want to be *seen*.

Date: June 13, 2013
Day of Week: Thursday
Time: 5:11 a.m.

TITLE OF DREAM/THEME: *The Visible Tree in the Field of Lavender*

PEOPLE/PLACES/THINGS: *Open field, tree*

FEELINGS/EMOTIONS: *(During or after waking) discomfort*

COLORS: *Lavender, green*

SYMBOLS: *Tree*

DETAILS: *I am in an open field of lavender with a single tree in view. I stand with my back against the tree. I look around and notice that the open field continues for miles around. There is a sense of discomfort. I wake up.*

INSPIRED ACTION STEPS/CHANGES/DECISIONS: *To explore the discomfort I felt in this dream*

Reflection: June 13, 2013, 8:05 P.M.

As I reflect on the image of the tree, what strikes me is how visible it is. There it stands in an open field to be seen from miles around, painting the sky with its branches and leaves. I imagine standing next to this tree, becoming imbued with the calming scent of lavender.

It is such beautiful scenery, yet a twinge of discomfort arises. It brings to mind a recurring theme from many of my childhood dreams. I had the ability to become invisible at will, either to escape a home invader or so I could explore a particular place without being seen. Being invisible offered a sense of protection. It felt safe.

How does this relate to my present reality? I recognize that I am a work in progress like everyone else. I'm stepping out and venturing into something new. Of course, remnants of old fears and hidden beliefs will surface when I am ready to deal with them. Now that I understand the root of this sensation, I can work at releasing old patterns that hinder me from moving forward with greater ease.

Once again, I return to the open field. My eyes are closed, feet firmly planted, arms outstretched. I am ready to step out without caring whether anyone is watching. I am clear about my intention. It is to be a conduit of love and compassion. I affirm that I am divinely embraced and guided. I accept the flow of my life and know that in this moment, I am safe.

A dream of hiding can also be seen as a message to honor your emerging self. You are a dynamic being, always in the process of growing and evolving. At times, you need space and solitude to hear yourself more clearly, to be more intentional about your next steps. Allow yourself the space, the stillness, the compassion to become who you aspire to be. When you are ready, come out of hiding and allow yourself to be seen.

RUNNING IN DREAMS

Unless you are an athlete or training for a marathon, a dream of running is often viewed as a sign of feeling overwhelmed and anxiety in your waking life. Typically, you run to evade an attacker or to avoid a threat to your physical well-being. You might metaphorically be running away from the overwhelming challenges you currently face. As your brain continues to keep you safely immobilized in bed, your dreaming mind might invent quicksand or other obstacles to account for your lack of forward movement, heightening the feelings of anxiety and fear.

If you were to consider the different stages in life, a dream of running could take on varied interpretations. In childhood, we prioritize self-preservation and instinctively run away from monsters, those known to us and those we invent in our creative minds. In adolescence, a time when we assert our independence, we metaphorically run from our childhood homes and from anything that attempts to confine us—and we run toward freedom, toward someone or something that fills our desire for connection and acceptance. In adulthood, we run to escape threats, real or perceived. We run without realizing that we are often running from ourselves.

Running depicts movement. If you adopt the perspective that dreams are constantly leading you toward healing and transformation, then there are more questions to be asked. It is not solely a question of *What are you running away from*, but also *What are you running toward?* What is life moving you toward? It is not enough to simply turn around and face the threat or to begin chasing after it. Instead, stop for a moment and consider the threat—who or what is it? Whatever it is—person, event, thing—invite it to be physically close to you in your waking imagination or if your dream state permits. What does it represent in you? What is its message to you? If it is, for example, a lion, it may be an invitation for you to witness another level of courage within yourself. Maybe the giant hawk swooping down intends no harm but desires your full attention. It takes courage to take a hawkeyed view of yourself, particularly when it comes to the areas of your life that would benefit from change.

Remember that the best in you is always in pursuit of you, but it never intends to scare you into vigilance or cause you to run away or hide. The invitation is always to stand in your integrity and return to the essence of who you are, who you have always been, and who you will always be, a child created from a love that transcends our limited physical expression of love.

FALLING IN DREAMS

The sensation of falling in dreams can be explained by the physiological changes that occur as we descend into the stages of sleep. In stage 1, your bodily processes begin to slow. Muscles relax with an occasional twitch, brain waves and eye movement become slower, and your heart rate drops. You begin to shift in and out of consciousness before fully disengaging from the external world and descending into subsequent stages of sleep. In stage 2, you drift further into non–rapid eye movement (NREM) sleep. This stage is characterized by lowered body temperature and short bursts of brain activity, allowing for minimal awareness of the external environment. If you feel that you never fully got to sleep, it is because you remained in this stage throughout most of the night. In stages 3 and 4, the brain experiences deeper states of sleep. This is where your blood pressure is lowest, you are less responsive to noise, and your body begins to repair and regenerate. In stage 5, you transition into REM sleep, where most dreaming occurs.

Gaiya, a 17-year-old student, shared that as she was falling asleep at about 1 A.M. she felt as though she was falling backward. She also expressed that it felt as though she had forgotten how to breathe, which was scary for her. Your body will not forget how to breathe, I assured her. The sensation of falling could also be related to an inner ear disturbance, affecting how movement is perceived. And particularly when we are extremely tired and drifting into sleep, the changing states in our body and brain can cause us to experience different sensations.

When the perception of falling occurs as you are dreaming, it is common to wake up before you hit the ground or other surface. Some people report hitting the surface then bouncing and floating. A common interpretation of falling in dreams is a sense of powerlessness, not having firm control in some aspect of life, work, finances, relationships, or physical or emotional well-being. Falling is often seen as failure. We fail to remain steady on our feet, to hold on to our sense of self, to succeed at pregnancy or parenthood, in friendship or marriage or at work. Things fall apart. However, what if falling is your inner being's way of surrendering? "If you can find grace or freedom in and through that falling," writes Richard Rohr in his book *Falling Upward*, "you find that it moves you forward, upward, broader, deeper, better—to growth."[2]

Falling can represent an invitation to begin anew. While trained gymnasts might land on their feet, some of us might have to sit or lie there for a while and observe the surroundings. Choosing to begin again does not mean that you know exactly what your next steps will be. It means that you are willing to continue on this grand adventure, trusting that in a universe that is so well organized, seemingly orchestrated at times, someday this too shall make sense. If you cannot immediately stand, begin by crawling. If you cannot lift yourself up, value yourself enough to call for help.

To fall in a dream might represent not a fall from safety but an opportunity to drop even deeper into all that you have the potential to be. What is your dreaming mind allowing you to see that you have been incapable of seeing about yourself? What are you falling toward? What greater purpose are you being asked to surrender to? What one gentle step will allow you to move in the direction to which you are being called?

FLYING IN DREAMS

Martin Luther King, Jr. is credited with saying, "If you can't fly, then run. If you can't run, then walk. If you can't walk, then crawl, but whatever you do, you have to keep moving forward."[3] Flying signifies the ultimate sense of achievement—freedom, autonomy, limitless possibility. We fly high, soaring to extraordinary heights, above the mountains and the clouds, capable of surmounting any earthly obstacle. "A bird may love a fish, signore, but where will they live?" asks Drew Barrymore's character in Andy Tennant's film *Ever After*. To which the portrayer of Leonardo da Vinci replies, "Then I shall have to make you wings."

In *Dreaming Gave Us Wings*, filmmaker Sophia Nahli Allison tells of the legend of enslaved Africans who could "fly" back home. She writes, "Rooted in the history of Igbo Landing—a site on Saint Simons Island, in Georgia, where enslaved people brought from Nigeria revolted and walked together into the marshy waters, rather than be sold into slavery—these stories became both a truth that enabled survival and an oral archive of resistance. Flight became a secret language for runaway slaves, and it continues to represent black mobility toward liberation."[4] To anyone with a history of enslavement or imprisonment, either physical or mental, flying in dreams represents a reclamation of dignity and a liberation not just of body or mind but also of soul.

Dreams of flying carry the message to reactivate your wings, your inner knowing that connects you to the infinite intelligence, the source of inspiration and all creation. To fly is to have steadfast hope, to recognize that freedom is not just an inalienable right; it is a divine inheritance bestowed at birth. It is not based on whether you are obedient or "good." No one deserves to be caged, shackled, or beaten into submission, either physically or emotionally. To dream of flying is not simply about your need to achieve lofty goals but to pursue whatever revitalizes you. It is not about escaping the challenges of this life but overcoming those challenges with grace and integrity. To fly is to free yourself from all that weighs you down: resentment, regret, past hurt, worry about the future. To fly is to encourage others to liberate themselves. But first: liberate yourself.

REMAINING GROUNDED IN THIS REALITY

Dreams are purposeful in serving the present reality. They reveal what is hidden, but in ways that honor the most vulnerable aspects of who you are. How? The ancient Egyptians would credit divine inspiration. Psychologist Carl Jung would say that a collaboration between the deep subconscious and higher regions of the brain occurs while we sleep. My discerning mind often wonders, *Was my dream a remnant of a stored childhood memory? If so, why has it now surfaced, seemingly unprovoked?* Once you commit to transformative healing, all aspects of your being become aware of this worthwhile intention. Similar to the neurons and chemical messengers that form networks of communication throughout your physical body, dreams assist in uncovering the root cause of fear and trauma responses. Through dream images, the unconscious can become conscious. What was once imperceptible can be perceived. All aspects of your being are involved in the process of healing.

Your dreams are an expression of all facets of your human experience—what is real, imagined, and yet to be realized. Your rebellious self, your adventurous self, your humorous self, your creative self, your doubtful self, your wounded self, your divine self—all can influence your dream imagery. You might find yourself doing something dangerous or objectionable in a dream that you would never do in reality, or something seemingly impossible, or even supernatural. Your dreaming mind knows no limits. It shows you unbridled possibilities and often circumvents the laws of this current reality, laws that are fundamental to how we relate to the physical world around us. For example, the law of gravity is often suspended in dreams. If you become lucid and recognize that you are dreaming, try jumping a few times in quick succession. You will likely begin to bounce and perhaps float.

Though your dreams might give you glimpses of other realities, you incarnated into this specific time in Earth's evolving story. It is essential that you remain grounded in this embodied reality. You are here not just to fulfill a single purpose but to exist purposefully. As you allow your dreams to reveal and guide, recognize that your level of critical awareness diminishes in dream states. You must confer with your rational mind in order to realize your highest potential. Rather than demonize your egoic tendencies, allow your rational mind to serve the best in you, your strengths, your passions, your authentic expression. Your dream world, your waking life, your family history, your personal history, your nation's history—while it all impacts how you exist in this reality, what matters most is that you decide to exist fully in the here and now.

UNDERSTANDING YOURSELF IN DEPTH

As Albert Einstein is often quoted as saying, "We have created a society that honors the servant [the rational mind] and has forgotten the gift [the intuitive mind]."[5] In earlier times, trained seers were revered for the insightful guidance they provided to the community. It was commonplace in many cultures to share dreams in a circle, where everyone gained valuable understanding of the world around them and everything in it. How did we get so far away from these practices? Did the "chosen" seers eventually misuse their power? Were our ancestors dispossessed of their gifts? Did communal laws and regulations override the importance of following one's inner moral compass?

While decorating gingerbread houses with other families one evening, a young boy said to me, "My mind says I want to eat more candy, but my heart says no. I don't know what to do." "Yes, you do," I answered. "Always follow your heart." How did he know the difference? Even the youngest among us can have an adept internal guiding system. Each time that guidance is affirmed, it strengthens. The wisest of teachers and healers will provide accessible tools, conventional and nontraditional methods, everything within their means that could be helpful to your overall well-being. They will seek to guide you inward, allowing you to recognize your inherent healing ability. Rather than dictate answers, they will provide questions that help you uncover all that you are.

When it comes to understanding yourself in depth, your dreaming eyes ask that you see from a wider perspective. With inner vision, you can observe your perceived shadows as unrealized potential. Your dreaming ears allow you to hear your innermost thoughts while no one is judging, including you. Your dreaming brain makes connections you would not ordinarily make while you are awake. You are not fully yourself when you are dreaming, but as a result of exploring your dream world, you can become more fully yourself once you awaken. You have the capacity to learn, grow, and understand the deepest aspects of yourself. As you learn to embrace all that you are, you can more easily determine how best to move through this complex world we call home.

HELPFUL QUESTIONS TO ASK YOUR DREAMS

First, understand that there is no one right question and no one right answer. Listen to all that emerges from within. Give space to all voices that are willing to speak.

1. What does this dream image or action (hiding, running, falling, flying, cooking, dancing, making love, etc.) represent in my current reality?

2. What specific area of my life (home, relationship, work, finances, mission, or aspect of myself—emotional, physical, mental, spiritual) needs my focused attention?

3. What aspect of myself is feeling difficult to embrace right now?

4. What is my dream calling me toward or away from?

5. How can I experience a greater sense of freedom and inner comfort in my waking life?

6. What else does my deepest wisdom want me to know?

DREAM VISUALIZATION PRACTICE FIVE: RECONNECTING WITH YOUR SHADOW SELF

Dreamscape: You are led through an untamed forest bursting with life to a clearing along a river's edge. Just as a forest embraces the visible and less visible inhabitants, you come face-to-face with an aspect of your shadow self. You are invited to embrace this shadow. Then, you hear the whisperings of your ancestors.

Objective(s): Inspired by the wisdom of Carl Jung, this practice encourages a compassionate view of our shadows, of all that we might feel ashamed of and attempt to suppress in order to fit in or be seen by others in a certain light. Learning to embrace all aspects of who you are is important for living a fully embodied and awakened life.

This practice is best done earlier in the evening to allow yourself time before bed to process any emotions and insights that might surface.

Visualization: As we ready ourselves for this healing practice, let us be fully grounded and centered in ourselves.

I invite you to adopt an open posture, sitting upright with your chest slightly lifted and your shoulders gently rolled back, palms resting on your lap or on your knees. Feel your body fully supported by the chair or by the floor.

I invite you to maintain this open posture as you place one hand on your heart. Inhale, receiving a nourishing breath into your heart, deep into your belly, and exhale.

Again, breathe deeply in through your heart, deep into your belly, and out through your heart.

Breathe deeply and release.

As you take another breath in, visualize this deeply nourishing breath traveling throughout your body, entering every organ, every tissue, every cell in your body before being released through the heart.

Continue to breathe as you find a rhythm that works best for you. You might keep your hand on your heart or place it back on your lap, whichever feels most comfortable.

Now imagine yourself walking through a forest bursting with life. Know that you are safe, that you are guarded, that you are protected.

The forest embraces its inhabitants. Take a moment to notice what is less visible. Notice the decaying leaves as well as the wildflowers, the pine needles as well as the pine cones. Notice the dark, moss-covered places. Notice the spaces between the leaves as the sunlight filters through the trees. Notice a caterpillar inching along a fallen branch. Just *notice*.

Breathe in the cool mountain air, feel the soft gentle breeze, and hear the birds as they call to each other. Listen as you continue on this path. You are never alone when you are among the trees, as the trees hold the breath of our ancestors. Listen for what they have to say.

Now imagine yourself coming upon a clearing at the edge of a river. See the mountains in the distance, hear the soothing sounds of the water, feel the warmth of the sun's rays.

Here at the river's edge, you come face-to-face with a reflection of you—your shadow. Through the lens of compassion, what do you say to your shadow self? What does your shadow say to you?

What words of wisdom might an ancestor or a wise elder offer to you?

I offer you these words. You might say to your shadow:

I see you. I see all that you are and all that you desire to be. I see you when you doubt yourself, your worth, your next steps. I see you when you question your wounds and when you feel ashamed of your scars. I see you when you're impatient, critical, feeling lonely and confused. And yet I see the essence of who you are, and who you have always been. I see you.

And your shadow might respond:

I hear you. I've heard your cries for our burdens to be lighter than they have been. I hear your desire to be released from the pain and the struggle, the fear and the uncertainty, to rise beyond the perceived darkness and exist more fully, not less. I hear your call for comfort and for greater ease. I hear you.

An ancestor might whisper through the trees:

I love you. I love and accept who you are and all that you have yet to become, the unfinished parts of you, which are the unfinished parts of me. I love how you keep learning and growing and becoming. I love you yesterday, today, and for all the tomorrows. I love you.

How would it feel to now embrace your shadow and have your shadow embrace you? When we embrace all aspects of ourselves, we exist more fully.

Embodiment: I invite you to slowly return to your breath, returning to the present time and space. Gently move and stretch your body, feeling your feet on the floor. When you are ready, open your eyes.

Now take some time to record this experience. Write down everything you wish to say to your shadow self, what your shadow self might say to you, and the wisdom offered to you by an ancestor or wise elder.

Return to this practice whenever you need to. See your life through the lens of compassion, rather than perfection. See each unfolding day as another opportunity to create, to love, to connect, to grow in acceptance of life's inevitable changes. Embrace all aspects of who you are and experience a greater sense of aliveness.

Chapter 5

RE-VISIONING "NIGHTMARES"

We had every intention of following through with a third attempt at gestational surrogacy. All of a sudden— or so it seemed—we were approaching two years since the second transfer. My husband was the one to broach the subject one evening. The more we talked, the more it became clear that neither of us truly wanted to proceed with another pregnancy attempt through surrogacy. After everything we had been through, it now seemed daunting. My friend, our gestational surrogate, understood. She generously gave us permission to change our minds. We all felt at peace with this decision.

As I journaled that evening, April 10, 2013, I recalled a dream of my grandmother from a month before.

March 2, 2013: *I am sitting in a living room with Mama. She shows me a photo of a white dove. In the photo, the dove flies for a few seconds, then stops. She shows me a second photo. Again, it is of a white dove that takes flight for seconds then stops. She is about to show me a third photo when someone else enters the room. Instead of showing me the third photo, she looks at me and shakes her head to indicate no.*

I had not connected this dream to the surrogacy when it occurred. I remember being fascinated that the dove became animated in the photo. When she shook her head, my initial interpretation was that this was just a special moment with her, a visitation not intended to be shared with anyone else. However, as I reread my dream journal entry, I wondered if this is what my inner being through the image of my grandmother was trying to communicate to me—that a third attempt would result in the same outcome.

It was not until September 2013 that I received a phone call from the clinic in reference to the continued storage of the frozen embryo. As I remember, it was a brief call. I expressed to the caller our decision not to continue with the surrogacy process, and vaguely remember her saying that the embryo would be discarded. I hung up the phone and was overcome by emotion. At the time of the call, I had been standing with my friend who had been our gestational surrogate, along with one of our neighbors. I had stepped away to take the call but was close enough that they were able to witness my tears.

A few weeks after the call from the fertility clinic, my dreaming mind apparently linked that phone conversation with another conversation, one I had with my daughter, one I can still easily recall. "I feel like I've lost someone," she said to me one evening at bedtime. It was the beginning of fourth grade, a new school in a new town. "You're probably missing your friends from your old school," I concluded. "No, Mom," she said, "it feels like it's someone from my family, but I don't know who it is." Those were her exact words. A comforting hug is all I could offer.

Days after, I woke from an imageless dream. With a racing heart and a sense of panic, it was as though my daughter's words, "No, Mom, it feels like someone from my family . . ." had instantly collided with the words spoken by the caller from the fertility clinic, "The embryo will be discarded." While I remembered hearing these words, their meaning did not register in that moment. I had relayed the details of the call to my husband, yet I have no memory of that conversation either. My daughter's words, however, continued to weigh on my mind.

My heart was consumed with regret that morning. My journal entry was just a series of questions—questions I would likely have asked had I been completely present in that phone call. Were there other options for us to consider, like possibly donating the frozen embryo to another infertile couple? While I cannot say for sure I would have considered that option, it did not occur to me before that moment of regret. In hindsight, it just seems like too important a decision to have been made over the phone without counsel. The voice of regret continued to ask impossible questions: How could she know that I was really who I said I was? How could she know that I would not later change my mind? Why had this been our decision to make? Why did I even answer the phone?

The following night, I awoke from another distressing dream. This time there was the image of a blue jay in a cage. It was squawking and flying about, continually hitting the sides of the cage as though it wanted to be released. I sat on the edge of the bed for a few minutes, but I was too awake to fall back to sleep. Instead, I left my bed and decided to do some focused breathing with my eyes closed. I visualized the cage to be on the floor of my living room. I saw a hand unlatching the cage and then imagined a woman's voice singing to this bird. I imagined the blue jay becoming less distressed before making its way out of the cage. It flew out of the cage, but then sat on top of the kitchen table for just a few seconds before making its way out through the sliding door in my kitchen. This imagery was soothing to my nervous system, and I was able to go back to bed and fall asleep. This dream and the re-visioning meditation inspired me to ceremoniously say good-bye to what now felt to be more than just a cluster of cells. Here is what I wrote in my journal on the evening of that day:

> September 25, 2013: *Tonight I light this candle. I open my heart and set this encapsulated energy free. You are more than a thought, more than an unrealized dream. You are more than a cluster of cells. You are a spark of creation, a tender piece of my heart. As you return to Spirit, I will rest in the peaceful knowing that energy can never by destroyed.*

While some nightmares are projections of disturbing images we might have heard about or seen on television or a movie screen, they all show us the creative power of our imagination and our brain's ability to replicate certain images and manufacture others. Nightmares allow us to see the power of our thoughts, beliefs, and brain chemistry in creating those images. They also serve to highlight information that may not be fully apparent to the conscious mind, information that we sometimes knowingly or unknowingly attempt to avoid, deny, or minimize. Nightmares indicate a sense of urgency. The terror we feel when we awaken from a frightening dream amplifies the message to reassess our current waking reality, to make changes when necessary. They often indicate that now is the time to address long-held fears, bottled-up grief, and other unresolved emotions that have found their way to the surface.

It is not that our inner being wishes to scare and further traumatize us. Nightmares come from all aspects of our inner world. They inform us that our conscious participation is required in order to fully heal—to no longer be silent, but to yell and scream and be comforted. A nightmare can also reveal possible ways to address overwhelming emotions such as fear and regret. While the dream of the blue jay was disturbing, it did offer a helpful suggestion that brought some resolution to the distress I had been experiencing, allowing me to live this day forward, choosing to let past decisions be what they were, serving as wisdom to guide future decision-making and greater compassion for myself and others.

DREAMING THE DREAM FORWARD

Once you understand that dreams serve as messengers, even the ones that you find terrifying can illuminate ways to transform your waking life. The practice of dreaming the dream forward is an empowering response to terrifying images and recurring nightmares. It recognizes your creative ability to imagine a different direction and ending to a disturbing dream. It helps you know that your dreams are a safe place to meet your self-doubt, anxiety, and other emotions. If you feel safe and grounded enough to do so, you can allow yourself to recall the imagery from the nightmare and create alternate pictures in your mind. Try inviting others into your dream landscape. This can be a loving presence from your current reality, a divine being, a religious figure, an animal guide, or a guardian. If you sense that a dream is linked to severe trauma, consider seeking professional help so that you can be guided appropriately.

In re-visioning a dream, you might also imagine yourself with traits or qualities that allow you to alleviate the distress that your dreaming mind conjures up. You are working with your imagination, so this can be anything you choose. If you have difficulty with visualization, prefer writing, or choose to do both, write out the dream with your preferred changes and the alternate ending of your choosing. Emotionally intense dreams tend to be easier to remember, so if you are able to go back to sleep after the dream you can wait until you are fully awake to re-vision the dream.

Dreaming the dream forward can also be done while you sleep. It was a high school classmate who shared this idea with me. Whenever he was having a scary dream, he would wake himself, then lie there and plan his next move. He would often reenter the dream where it left off and was able to enact his plan. The awareness of *this is a dream* can also trigger lucidity. With the knowing that you are dreaming as you are dreaming, you can intentionally direct the events of your dream in an even more elaborate way.

SLEEP PARALYSIS

Sleep paralysis—the sensation of being awake yet not being able to move or communicate though you have a clear sense of your surroundings—occurs while transitioning into and out of sleep. It can be frightening. Some people describe the experience of sensing the presence of another person or something else in the room, which layers on the fear that the entity is either choosing not to help or that the dreamer simply cannot communicate that they need help. There are also reports of feeling as though they are being suffocated. The word *nightmare* is derived from an old belief that a threatening spirit would sit on the chest of the dreamer, rendering them unable to move and causing disturbing dreams.

Though worrisome, you are not in danger of being suffocated by a ghostly intruder or "evil" entity when this occurs. The temporary inability to move your muscles is your body's way of keeping you and others safe by preventing you from acting out your dreams. Your ability to breathe and maintain other life-sustaining processes remain unaffected. Though sleep paralysis is common, particularly with erratic sleep patterns or sleeping on your back when you are moderately to severely exhausted, some researchers cite medication use and sleep disorders such as sleep apnea and narcolepsy as possible underlying causes.

Dr. Clare Johnson, a renowned expert in lucid dreaming, argues that sleep paralysis can also be used as a "springboard" into lucid dream experiences. After hearing Dr. Johnson speak, I decided to put this to the test. When I experienced an episode of sleep paralysis, I immediately recalled her guidance. Instead of struggling to wake myself or groan so my husband could wake me, I remained calm and observed what was happening. There were no images—just darkness and the awareness of my bedroom. I felt the sensation of floating upward to the ceiling then back down onto my bed. Remaining calm was key to waking more effortlessly from this uncomfortable dream state.

HYPNAGOGIC AND HYPNOPOMPIC HALLUCINATIONS

Hypnagogia and hypnopompia are transitional states of consciousness between wakefulness and sleep. Hypnopompia occurs as we transition from sleep to waking, while hypnagogia is the transitional period occurring as we drift into sleep. In either of these states, it is possible to imagine sensations, smells, sounds, and visual images not perceived by others. These illusory experiences can be associated with sleep disorders such as narcolepsy or with anything that impacts brain chemistry like drug use or alcohol consumption. They can also occur during periods of sleep deprivation, elevated stress, and anxiety. And yet these states of consciousness are what have gifted writers, artists, and inventors with extraordinary insights and creations.

When faced with a complex problem, inventor Thomas Edison was known to nap holding a steel ball in each hand. Just on the edge of sleep as his muscles relaxed, the balls would fall onto metal saucers, startling Edison awake from the hypnagogic state. He would then record any thoughts or images he could recall, which often led to solutions that were not accessible when he was wide awake. Many others have reported waking in the hypnopompic state with an original plot for a novel, a creative solution, or other innovation.

Psychologist Vaughan Bell wrote this about hypnagogia in *The Atlantic*:

> *"It is brief and often slips by unnoticed, but consistent careful attention to your inner experience after you bed down can reveal an unfolding mindscape of curious sounds, abstract scenery, and tumbling thoughts."*[1]

This "unfolding mindscape" as Bell describes can be used to reprogram our subconscious mind as we drift to sleep. Affirmations such as "It is safe to fall asleep" or "I am safe, guarded, and protected" can be soothing to the nervous system. Like dreaming the dream forward, you might invite a reassuring presence or guardian to keep a watchful eye. You might find a unique way to stave off scary images. Marlia, a woman in her 20s, loves to watch horror movies at night but she of course does not enjoy when these images reappear as she is falling asleep. Her solution? Right before she falls asleep, she allows herself to remember the scariest scenes and then imagines them being erased as you would erase a blackboard. The empty blackboard is the last thing she sees before falling asleep.

One common hypnopompic hallucination is hearing your name being called. You might even have responded verbally to this seemingly real and familiar voice only to find that it was just an auditory hallucination. You are usually startled awake at exactly the time you knew you needed to wake up. In that case, your inner wisdom collaborated with your brain and woke you up at just the right time.

FALSE AWAKENINGS

One patient shared her experience of false awakenings. She would experience waking up, getting ready for work, and getting into her car before realizing that she was still in bed and had been dreaming. She would then get out bed, shower, and get dressed only to wake up again. In a false awakening, the person is unaware that they are dreaming, and the same scene might repeat several times before they actually awaken. This is due to the familiarity of the environment and routine nature of daily tasks that are featured in these types of dreams. Whatever we repeatedly do in the daytime can become what we also dream we are doing. Fortunately, muscle atonia typically keeps us safe in bed while dreaming. Though our minds are active, our bodies are physiologically asleep.

My patient shared that her experience of false awakenings was happening at a time in her life when she was overly stressed and often physically and emotionally exhausted by the time she went to bed. Even after hearing her alarm clock and confident that she was fully awake, she still felt uneasy about the frequency of these occurrences. She then took a mindfulness course that provided techniques that helped to manage her stress, and the false awakenings eventually stopped.

Another strategy to determine when you are dreaming is to practice what are known as "reality checks." Lucid dreaming teacher and author Charlie Morley recommends simply looking at your hand throughout the day, flipping it over, and then flipping it back to see if anything changes. You will notice that nothing changes. However, in a dream state where the brain is more creative, you might flip your hand back over to find that something has appeared in your hand, or that five fingers have become seven. As Morley explains to his students, "When we ask the brain to maintain the projection of a particular image or replicate the exact scene, the brain will produce a close but imperfect replication."[2] If we practice this in our waking states, this level of awareness can enter our dream states. An example of this is a dream I had of waking up and walking through my house late at night, noticing I had left certain lights on. As I attempted to turn off the lights, I was unable to move my arm. I could see the light switch, but I could not lift my arm. I started to think that something was seriously wrong. Then other lights started to turn on. The thought entered my dreaming mind that this could be a dream and I had the awareness to look down at my hands. Sure enough, all the lights instantly turned off. I woke up to find that I was still in bed, lying on my right arm, which had fallen asleep.

4 BEDTIME PRACTICES TO SOOTHE THE NERVOUS SYSTEM

If you can maintain the awareness to remain calm in your dream states, even scary images can be less threatening. To do this, create a consistent daytime practice and bedtime routine that are soothing to the nervous system. Here are four simple practices you might wish to incorporate.

1. Breathing into Your Heart

Heart-centered breathing as taught by HeartMath Institute has been found to regulate the nervous system. It integrates the intelligence of the heart, mind, and body. Lie comfortably in bed with a pillow under your knees to support your back. Place one hand on the center of your chest. Place the other hand on your belly. As you breathe deeply, imagine each breath being received into the heart, traveling down into the belly. As you exhale, imagine the breath traveling up from the belly and exiting the heart. Breathe in peace. Breathe out peace.

2. Frontal-Occipital Holding

This technique is based on cranial osteopathy and the work of Dr. William Sutherland. It is also known as emotional stress release (ESR), as it induces a relaxation response throughout your body. Lie comfortably on your back, supporting your head and your knees with a pillow. Gently place the palm of one hand on your forehead. Place your other hand on the lowest part of the back of your head. Hold this position as you focus on a specific thought—any thought, even one that is worrisome—or allow your mind to wander. You can also visualize a calming scene or state an affirmation like "It is safe for me to fall asleep." Deepen the relaxation response with slow, deep breaths. Continue to cradle your head for as long as you need.

3. Practicing Self-Forgiveness

Take a moment each night to practice self-forgiveness. This life is a series of unique experiences that you have never lived before. Give yourself permission to be who you were on your way to becoming who you are now and accept who you will become next. Practicing self-forgiveness allows you to make choices that align with your present self, rather than who you used to be.

If a moment of regret comes to mind, send a blessing of love to that experience. Allow it to serve as wisdom as you move forward with the intention of living more fully aligned with the person you desire to become.

4. Practicing Surrender

This practice also allows you to surrender concerns or regrets to the larger wholeness, the source of all creation that organizes and supports this reality. Assume a comfortable position in bed with support pillows in place. Place your arms at your side, palms facing up. Whenever worrisome or anxious thoughts enter your mind, visualize them as a flow of energy, moving from your head, traveling down your arms, and into your hands. Now allow this energy to flow out of your hands and into the hands of grace, trusting in the love and wisdom that is within us and beyond us. Feel your body soften and relax, knowing that a restorative night's sleep will allow for greater clarity and creative solutions to the challenges you face. Breathe in love. Breathe out love. Breathe in gratitude. Breathe out gratitude. Rest.

STEPS FOR RE-VISIONING A NIGHTMARE

1. First and foremost, know that you are safe. Whatever is happening in your mind is happening only in your mind.

2. Use frontal-occipital holding or another technique to become calm and regulate your nervous system. If you are immediately able to fall back to sleep, allow yourself to do so, and know that it is safe.

3. Remember that you are the ultimate creative director of your inner world. Consider why you had this dream. What are you being asked to acknowledge, process, and heal in your waking life? What fears do you need to address with compassion and honesty? Consider how aspects of this dream might

be guiding you to wholeness, connection, and purpose.

4. Envision a new direction or dream ending whenever possible. Choose life. Choose freedom. Choose love.

DREAM VISUALIZATION PRACTICE: MEETING YOUR INNER CREATIVE MUSE

Dreamscape: You are in a dimly lit room, seated in front of a cozy fire. Here you will meet and engage with your inner creative muse, the part of you that connects your stored thoughts, memories, and other imagery to create your dream narratives. You will observe and listen without judgment.

Objective(s): To engage with varying aspects of yourself and observe what connections arise in your waking state; this helps you see how your inner creative muse seamlessly connects your thoughts and memories while you sleep.

Visualization: You are seated in a comfortable chair, with your favorite blanket in front of a cozy fire. Feel the warmth of the flames and relax into this present moment, closing your eyes if you like.

Breathe in deeply through the nose. Exhale slowly, releasing all the tension in your body.

Breathe in, breathe out. Breathe in, breathe out.
Notice.
Notice any thoughts, images, or memories that spontaneously arise.
Observe.

Allow your inner creative muse to reveal itself to you in whatever form it chooses.

What might this image say?
Listen.
Listen without judgment, without expectation or attachment, but with a desire for truth.
Listen with openness, with serenity, with courage.
Listen for guidance.
Listen for insight.
What do you hear?

Now ask yourself these questions: *Who is this version of me in my dreams who knows me so intimately?*

See what arises.

Who is the me who knows the inner recesses of my heart, who knows what terrifies me and what motivates me?

What images or thoughts arise?

What is the aspect of myself that accepts me in my humanness and loves me unconditionally, even in moments when I feel I am unable to love and accept myself?

What thoughts or images arise?

Who is this being of grace, of mercy, of greater understanding who desires for me to exist more, not less?

Listen fully and completely.

Embodiment: When you are ready, slowly return to the present moment. Be aware of the room you are actually in. Feel your feet on the floor. Be conscious of your breath. When you are fully present, record the details of this experience, including any insights and guidance you received.

When we actively listen to our innermost thoughts and sort through our emotions, we are less likely to experience terrifying dreams that are determined to get our attention.

Chapter 6

DREAM PLAY AND EXCAVATING YOUR INNATE GIFTS

Over the years I have received gifts of jade in the form of bracelets, pendants, and loose gemstones. These were precious reminders that though I had given birth to a child no one else knew and loved as I did, I was not alone in remembering her name. For others to acknowledge that she had existed in this time and space meant so much. There was also a greater feeling of calm whenever I wore the stone. When I wore jade, it felt as though I could breathe more effortlessly, more deeply, allowing for a greater sense of ease and clarity of mind. I would touch and massage the pendant on my necklace or mindlessly play with my bracelet and feel a tickling yet soothing sensation throughout my body—almost like feeling goose bumps when something resonates. One day a friend noticed my necklace and shared the benefits of this semiprecious stone. "What made you choose the name Jade?" she asked. "I feel as though it chose me," I heard myself say.

DREAM STONES

According to various sources, jade is a "dream stone," capable of bringing meaningful dreams and creative insights to the dreamer. It is also believed to enhance the ability to decode dreams. One night, while wearing a necklace with a jade pendant, I had this dream.

May 17, 2017: *Last night I dreamed of a young child who appeared to be alone on a beach. Though blind, she could see the sun's shadow. Evening after evening, she existed alone, knowing when the sun appeared by its shadow. She would then sit or lie down and stare at the sun's shadow until one day she began to see a little speck of light. The more she stared, the larger and brighter this little light became.*

Excitedly, she concentrated even more, focusing until she could no longer look at the sun. It was then that she was able to see fully. The sun's light had given her vision.

She looked around and saw barren land and water. And with such joy in her heart combined with the sun's light, her mind began to think in images and in color. Anything she could think of became manifest.

Up until that point, her only nourishment came through the soles of her bare feet, absorbing minerals and fluids from the earth, her mother. Harnessing the energy of her father, the sun, she continued to create. She created trees and flowers and fruit, the animals, and everything else around her.

She began to play even more with her abilities until she created a playmate in her image.

And since she had the ability to create, everything she created also had the ability to create.

The playmates could not see their own faces, only each other. The more of them that began to exist, the more creative they became in choosing different shapes, sizes, and colors.

How can certain stones and crystals influence dreams? As it is explained in the following quote attributed to Albert Einstein: "Match the frequency of the reality you want, and you cannot help but get that reality. It can be no other way. This is not philosophy. This is physics."[1] We are all receptors and transmitters of energy. Our thoughts, emotions, and words vibrate at varying frequencies, impacting how we view and respond to the world around us. Everything has an energetic frequency—our food, the trees, the plants, the ground we walk upon, and inanimate objects. How we interact with these energies determines our mental, emotional, and physical health, and it impacts the natural world. Indigenous practices from multiple countries remind us that reciprocity is fundamental to our relationship to everything that exists around us. We are to take only what is needed and always give something in return. As we tend to the needs of the earth, our needs are also tended.

Eliot Cowan, author of *Plant Spirit Medicine*, invites us to approach everything in the natural world with interest and respect rather than belief or disbelief. There is wisdom yet to be gathered and integrated from the natural elements that have existed long before our human ancestors. Gems and stones have existed beneath the earth's surface for billions of years. Imagine the transformations they have undergone and all they have witnessed. Imagine the stories they would tell if they could. Cowan states, "By leaning toward the question of 'what would happen if I were to approach life as an inquisitive seeker,' we can begin to rediscover the essence and vast possibilities of all aspects of life that lie in wait around us."[2] What if we applied this approach not only to our waking lives but also to our dream states?

The concept of dream play allows for enhanced dream experiences by relying on the power of the mind, intention, and our ability to suspend our disbelief, as articulated by renowned spiritual teacher Dr. Wayne Dyer. In other words, we make ourselves available to what is not yet seen or known. We practice letting go of all that might seem unlikely or impossible. We remain open to possibility—the possibility of being guided to our fullest potential. We may not understand how or why, but we allow for the experience. We allow for the invisible to become visible, for the undiscovered to be discovered.

For thousands of years, natural elements like crystals have been used as tools to support the physical, emotional, and spiritual well-being of humans. The success of these healing methods implies that we are inherently connected to nature. We are not just on this earth; we are *of* this earth. Still, we each have a unique constitution that determines how we perceive the varied energies we are exposed to. This means that what benefits one may not benefit all. Nature teaches us that diversity is essential to our continual evolution.

You can place a stone, a photo of a loved one, or other memorabilia under your pillow, under your bed, or at your bedside to safely influence sleep and dreams. To help you get started, here are seven common dream stones and their reported effects.

Amethyst

Amethyst is known to magnify energy and promote vivid dreaming. However, if someone is more energetically sensitive, it could prevent them from having a restful night's sleep.

Celestite
Celestite is a calming stone that helps dreamers remember their nightly dreams. It is also considered to be one of the best stones for restful sleep.

Dream Quartz
Dream quartz is also known as lodolite, garden quartz, or the shaman's stone. It is a rare stone that is used by shamans for vision quests. It is also believed to enhance dream recall and lucid dreaming.

Hematite
Hematite is a grounding stone that helps you remain asleep, allowing for longer periods of dreaming sleep.

Jade
Though commonly found in shades of green, jade comes in a wide variety of colors. Blue jade can be used to calm the mind, promote visions, assist in remembering dreams, and enhance lucid dreaming.

Moonstone
Moonstone is believed to stimulate the pineal gland and the release of melatonin, a key hormone that regulates sleep. It has a gentle energy that supports restful sleep and dreaming.

Quartz
Quartz, or clear quartz, is known for its harmonizing effects on the body and mind, along with its

ability to maintain precise frequencies. It is often used to set powerful intentions.

3 TIPS FOR WORKING WITH CRYSTALS AND STONES

1. Be Intentional

Intend to choose a stone that is intent on choosing you. As Cowan and other Indigenous healers recommend, see the stone as an entity deserving of honor and respect. Extend gratitude for its existence. Set a personal intention for what you want to experience with this stone. You might simply ask the stone to serve as a reminder to record your dreams when you awaken, or to prompt you to express gratitude every morning.

2. Cleanse and Recharge

Rituals are a sign of respect, honor, and intention. The ritual of cleansing and recharging removes and transmutes unwanted energies that the stone has already absorbed. This can be done by placing the stone in sunlight or moonlight for a recommended amount of time or burying it in a pot of fertile dirt. Be aware of inclement weather to avoid damage to the stone. Some softer stones can dissolve when exposed to or submerged in water. Direct sunlight or prolonged heat can also be damaging.

Certain crystals, such as quartz and selenite, can be used to cleanse and recharge other crystals. The crystals in need of recharging can be placed directly on top of a flat piece of selenite. The stone needing to be charged could also be encircled by pieces of quartz, salt, or other charged crystals.

Using sage or smudging is another way of cleansing a stone. In a well-ventilated room, light a smudge stick made of white sage leaves and twine. Once it begins to create smoke, you can pass each gemstone through the smoke. A mist made of sage essential oils can also be used when burning sage is not appropriate.

It is recommended that crystal and stones be cleansed before initial use, after being worn, or if handled by another person. They can also be cleansed and recharged weekly or monthly. Trust your intuitive sense, as it will know exactly when to do so.

3. Expand Self-Awareness

Be aware of how your body responds in the presence of crystals or any other tools used to improve your well-being. Take note of subtle changes, like your ability to take deeper breaths. Notice how you feel when the stone is nearby versus when it is farther away. If you find yourself tossing and turning in bed for no apparent reason, you might want to try moving the crystal a distance away or to another room. How does it feel when you hold the stone, or when it is worn as a bracelet or necklace? Body awareness is an important practice in helping to conserve your energy reserves and minimizing undesirable affects. It allows you to know whenever anything or anyone invigorates or leaves you feeling depleted. It is empowering to align with energies that are life-affirming.

RHYTHMIC BEATS

Another tool I found soothing after losing Jade was the sound of drums. The rhythmic beats echoed the sound of her heartbeat I would listen for during ultrasound visits, and they brought comfort when silence seemed unbearable. The vibrations counteracted the numbing effects of grief. I soon noticed that the sounds and vibrations not only lulled me to sleep but seemed to somehow transport me into other states of consciousness. I would often emerge with a greater sense of peace, ready to face another day.

In her book *When the Drummers Were Women*, Layne Redmond tells of this forgotten aspect of women's heritage. A handheld frame drum was seen as a ritual instrument used by shamans and seers—primarily women—to connect with the earth's natural rhythms for healing and transformation. Redmond writes, "In the oldest cultures, rhythm was revered as the structuring force of life."[3] The drum was used to deepen individual and communal connection to ancient goddesses and priestesses. Redmond explains how our female ancestors were dispossessed of this spiritual heritage and invites us to now "resurrect the values once associated with female-based religious systems—values of compassion and healing, of providing and sheltering, of nourishing, of holding all life sacred."

Drumming can be used to restore a sense of harmony with the outer world and within ourselves. The rhythms invite us to fully inhabit the present moment. The vibrations calm and regulate areas of the brain and nervous system. This present-moment awareness and balanced emotional state are essential to restful sleep, dreaming, and living through our most challenging days. Robert Lawrence Friedman, author of *The Healing Power of the Drum*, led a drumming circle for the community of Newtown, Connecticut, after the 2012 tragedy at Sandy Hook Elementary School. The participants were able to express and release the energy of their emotions without having to "find the right words." When words are not adequate, rhythmic beats can help to release sadness, anger, and other felt emotions.

Whether you listen to drumming, purchase your own frame drum, or participate in a drumming circle or other sound therapy, rhythmic beats can be beneficial in many ways. Researchers have verified that the rhythmic energy transmitted through drumming synchronizes both hemispheres of the brain, allowing for the release of serotonin and hormones that improve mental clarity and optimism. The increase in alpha brain waves is also associated with increased creativity and deeper states of consciousness.[4]

IMAGINATION

Imagination allows you to bring a future dream into the present reality. The power of your imagination can place you anywhere you wish to be. It can return you to a memorable period in your life, one filled with exuberant fun, connection, and when your immediate world was filled with promise. Hold those images in your thoughts and your body will instantly create chemical changes, causing specific bodily reactions and sensations to arise. These moments, no matter how brief, can be just enough to turn up the level of joy when you might be experiencing hopelessness. Pay attention to the images you create and you will come to know that you are a co-creative being, capable of boundless growth.

Your dreaming mind can also make connections and take you to worlds that you have yet to imagine. You might experience colors and scenery that are beyond what you can recall ever seeing with your physical eyes. You might hear a melody or lyrics that have not yet been heard by anyone else. Nevertheless, you are the intended recipient, the one meant to bring that song into this reality so that it can be heard and enjoyed by others. "Yesterday," one of the most popular songs by the Beatles, came to band member Paul McCartney in a dream. He is quoted as saying, "That was entirely magical—I have no idea how I wrote that. I just woke up one morning and it was in my head. I didn't believe it for about two weeks."[5] Again, suspend your disbelief.

Just imagine the possible adventures our children could experience each night if they recognized the extent of their dreaming minds. Imagine if they were excited to get to bed each night with the possibility of reentering a fun dream they began the night before. What if they knew it was even possible to practice their skills as a gymnast, ball player, or swimmer? Lucid dreaming and mindfulness researcher Dr. Tadas Stumbrys published a peer-reviewed article in the *Journal of Sports Sciences* on this topic.[6] He and other esteemed researchers found that practicing motor skills while lucid dreaming improved skill performance just as effectively as actual physical practice of that sport or skill. This means that shooting a basketball or playing soccer in your dream could improve your abilities in these activities when awake.

AWAKENING TO YOUR INNATE GIFTS

Ultimately, when we grant ourselves permission to be intentional with our dreams, we begin to see our waking lives as opportunities to grow, create, and step fully into our true selves. André Rochais, an educator in the areas of personal growth, human relationships, and spiritual transformation once said, "Indeed, we are asleep on a treasure, on a wellspring of energy, on a volcano of creativity, and on incredible reserves of genuine love. Everything is here in the very heart of humanity, within the depths of men and women of this planet; everything necessary is here to forge a more human world."[7] How do we begin to unearth innate gifts that have been buried under decades of conditioning?

First, practice self-compassion. When it comes to spiritual growth, all-or-nothing is an unhelpful mindset. Not being exactly where you had hoped to be at the current stage of your life does not mean you have failed. It means that you are in progress. It might mean that you have been directed elsewhere. Everything you have ever experienced has gotten you to this point. You cannot simply separate the dark from the light as you would a pile of laundry. Every period of your life has contributed to the person you have become and the person you are becoming. Acknowledge that you could not have known then what you know now. Grant yourself permission to be flawed and unfinished in a world that often demands that you be flawless and complete.

Allow yourself adequate time to grow into who you wish to become. "There is more to learn," someone I admire greatly once said to me in a dream. It was not what I wanted to hear at the time, but it was necessary. We do not magically become who we desire to be without integrating all the lessons we have gathered along the way. Sometimes those lessons get repeated until we understand them more fully. It is no accident that we tend to teach what we most need to learn.

Date: November 9, 2012
Day of Week: Friday
Time: 6:20 a.m.

TITLE OF DREAM/THEME: *There Is More to Learn*

PEOPLE/PLACES/THINGS: *Cheryl, an auditorium, large crowd, a stage*

FEELINGS/EMOTIONS: *(During or after waking) Self-doubt, unprepared*

COLORS: *Gray*

SYMBOLS: *A stage, books*

DETAILS: *I am at a Hay House event, and I'm unexpectedly called to the stage as one of the speakers. Feeling unprepared, I hastily exit through the back. On my way out, I see Hay House author Cheryl Richardson sitting at a table preparing to sign her books. I approach her table and she immediately says to me, "There is more to learn."*

INSPIRED ACTION STEPS/CHANGES/DECISIONS:
Self-doubt allows me to take pause and be more discerning about my next steps in fulfilling my aspirations as an author and speaker.

There is always more to learn when you seek to become the most authentic expression of who you are. The road that leads you to where you can best serve is often long and winding. It is not intended to discourage, though. It is meant to strengthen your inner resolve, to prepare you for the reality that not everyone you meet upon the path will understand, agree with, or support your waking dreams. They might serve as mirrors, allowing you to see how far you have traveled. They might reveal that you still have some growing to do. We all do. Know that even in moments of self-doubt, your innermost voice is calling you to listen more deeply, to be more discerning. Attune to that voice within, even if surrounding voices are much louder. Take all the time you need for a soft yes to become a resounding YES. Likewise, it might require more growth and healing for you to accept that the answer is not the one you had expected.

On the other hand, do let yourself grieve for what could have been, for what you hoped might be. Understand that grief is not a linear process with an expiration date. Like everything, it can be cyclical or spontaneous. Treat it as you would any unexpected but well-known visitor; you would likely invite them in or at least listen to what they have to say.

> November 3, 2010: *Tears begin to well up in me as I think that I could never again safely carry a child. I knew this before now, but today it really sank in. It saddens me. It feels like a dream that was unrealized, a prayer that went unanswered. So now I must accept this reality that feels so heavy right now. At my core, I am a mother. This is what I was created for.*

Allow your inner wisdom to reveal what your conscious mind might be adept at hiding. Blame, shame, guilt, and regret must be recast or they will keep you anchored in the belief that the past could have been different. Blame is often disempowering because it places the responsibility of your continued well-being into the hands of another. Rather than blame, seek support from those who are willing and able. Though the power to transform comes from within, adequate support and guidance are always necessary. As for shame, guilt, and regret, they are painful but not intended to be paralyzing. Let them serve as wisdom, not prisons.

Recognize that everything is a teacher, that pain in all its forms is a thorough excavator, breaking us open, disturbing and exposing our depths. It is often in the depths of despair and uncertainty that we are able to access our incredible reserves—reserves of love, hope, faith, trust, generosity, and compassion. I have often wondered if I could have been who I am now without the pain, the struggle, the loss, the disappointments. I would still have been kind, but grief has tilled the soil of kindness and active compassion has emerged. This entire journey has cultivated faithfulness to the source of goodness and trust in my deeper wisdom. It has set me onto a path I may not have otherwise chosen, but I now know it is exactly where I am meant to be.

In gardening, some believe that no-till methods should be employed. No-till is based on the idea that soil should be disturbed as little as possible to reduce or prevent erosion. However, the process of tilling is a form of deep cultivation that prepares the ground for a new season of growth. Many of us gravitate toward comfort and certainty, and only when we experience discomfort do we begin to explore our deeper selves, or follow the trail where we are being led. Years ago, had anyone said to me that I would one day write a book that shared my personal story, my dreams, and journal entries, I would have confidently stated, "No way, that will never happen."

You will find your greatest gifts at the core of who you are. Life is always leading you there—not always in the ways you may prefer, but in ways that are often necessary. You may suffer greatly, but the need is to integrate all you have learned to excavate that which is held within you. Allow others to accompany you. Let yourself be helped, and in turn, help at least one other person. It will take the efforts of many to reduce and end the suffering of all. That is why the fullness of you is needed in this space and time. Your gifts are needed. How you decide to share these gifts, though, is still up to you. If the path is not yet clear, pause. Every journey requires a period of rest. The more sensitive you are, the more rest you need. And that is okay.

PREPARING FOR SLEEP

Bedtime practices are essential to ensure deep rest. Give yourself time to adequately prepare for bed by implementing self-care rituals such as a warm bath, a foot bath, or even a gradual dimming of the lights. Disconnect from screens and other electronic devices. Allow yourself to enter sleep with a sense that whatever is left undone today can be revisited tomorrow. Here are some helpful recommendations.

1. Spend a few moments before bed looking up at the night sky, either standing outside or looking out through a window. Notice the different stages of the moon—sometimes it is soft and blurred, sometimes bright and full. Notice the stars that you can easily see, and imagine the ones you cannot. Recognize that without the darkness, there cannot be light. Recognize that you are connected to a greater universe beyond what you alone can imagine.

2. Interact with a plant. Touch, provide water, and express gratitude for the plant. There is an interesting study by Wenzhu Zhang and his colleagues at the School of Biological Science and Medical Engineering at Beihang

University on the emotions and sleep of isolated individuals on deep-space missions and deep-sea explorations.[8] The study found that the fragrance and green color of plants helped to regulate emotions and improve sleep quality. Exposure to coriander plants allowed participants in the study to fall asleep quickly and sleep deeply. Strawberry plants were shown to improve the emotional state of participants because they are edible, not based on their fragrance.

3. Express appreciation for your physical body. We often drift asleep preoccupied with today's events and tomorrow's expectations without expressing gratitude for the vessel that allows us to express ourselves. Rest your hands anywhere on your body and spend a few moments giving thanks for each body part. Thank the ones that function optimally and the ones that need regeneration and repair. Thank your internal intelligence for conducting these processes while you sleep. In giving thanks to the body, we give thanks to the power that created the body.

DREAM VISUALIZATION PRACTICE: EXCAVATING YOUR INNATE GIFTS

Dreamscape: You are on an archaeological expedition where you explore a cave and unearth your hidden gifts.

Objective(s): To recognize our innate gifts that are meant to be embraced and shared with others

Visualization: With an open heart and mind, I invite you to sit comfortably.

Bring your attention to your breath, the breath of life that connects you to the source of all that is, the earth, to her trees and plants, her rocks and her gemstones. Breathe and connect to all of creation, the greater universe, all that is seen and unseen, all that is yet to be known.

Breathe deeply, receiving, being nourished,
being replenished.
Exhale slowly, returning the breath,
nourishing, replenishing.

Breathe deeply.
Exhale slowly.

Imagine yourself at the entrance of a cave. Who is with you on this expedition? It could be other versions of yourself, a trusted companion, or a guide. Perhaps you are alone. No matter what, you are safe. You are held. You are guided.

When you are ready, enter the cave. You are well-prepared. You have all you need and more. Allow your inner compass to light the way.

When you first enter the cave, notice carvings on the walls left behind by our ancestors.

They are the ones who have led you here, not solely because of their faith in you but also because they want you to have faith in yourself.

What symbols or words are written on the wall?

What message do they communicate?

I offer you this message . . .

Your truest essence is love. You are a creative being, constantly expanding and returning to all that you are. Seek to understand that storms naturally come and go, not to discourage or destroy but to alter the course when necessary. Know that you cannot give without receiving. In this ever-changing voyage of healing and becoming free, you are healed as you heal, you are set free as you liberate others. You are loved and you are love.

You are invited to go deeper into the cave.

When you arrive at the deepest part of the cave, you will know.

Here, your treasures lie.

Now you get to decide. Which gifts are you ready to receive? The gift of compassion? The gift of curiosity? The gift of creativity? The gift of determination? The gift of humor?

What is at the root of this gift? The love of community? The love of family? The love of adventure? Or simply love?

As you retrieve your gifts from this cave, leave something behind: a promise, words of gratitude, or both.

I offer you these promises . . .

I will take only what I need when I need it.
I will not overextend my resources or sacrifice my well-being.
I will seek to give when I feel restored, not when I feel depleted.

You might offer these words of gratitude . . .

Thank you to all my ancestors and guides, known and unknown. Thank you for your guidance, your wisdom, your love. Thank you for dreaming me into being. Thank you for holding my hand in yours. Thank you for leading me inward to where all my treasure awaits.

See yourself making your way out of the cave, back into this current time and space.

Embodiment: Return to your breath. Breathe deeply as you reinhabit this present moment. Gently begin to move about and stretch your body. I invite you to take some time to write about your experience of this practice.

What other messages did you retrieve from the walls of the cave? Which gift or gifts are you ready to inhabit more fully? How might you use these gifts in service, where you can best serve and be served?

May you know that you are a valuable part of an interconnected whole.
May you come to know your true value.
May you know that you are loved.
May you know peace.

PART II

RECOGNIZING THE INTERCON-NECTEDNESS OF ALL THAT IS

Chapter 7

A SEA OF ORDINARY
AND "BIG" DREAMS

"Go to the sea," my grandmother's words continue to echo. The sea is vast and unending. It is awe-inspiring and mysterious, powerful and unpredictable. "When we go back to the sea," said John F. Kennedy, ". . . we are going back from whence we came."[1] When we return to the sea, we are returning to the sea of creation, of possibility. It is here that we begin to recognize that human beings are not simply a part of the natural world; we *are* nature, and we express its intelligence and wonder. We are not merely walking upon this earth. She is our mother. She knows the sea intimately, not just what is visible on the surface but also what lies beneath. And when she sends us to the sea, it is so our hearts can glimpse the interconnectedness of all that is, seen and unseen, known and unknown.

In this way, dreams are much like the sea, mysterious and filled with possibility. Behind closed eyes, we enter a world of darkness. It is this darkness that restores our inner sight, our soul's vision. Dreams give us glimpses of what is not yet visible in our waking perception of life. They can construct an entirely new version of the world as we know it. In dreams, the rational mind remains a curious onlooker, the brain becomes masterfully creative, hidden emotions come out of hiding, and our innermost being poetically shares its wisdom through symbols and imagery.

ORDINARY DREAMS

An ordinary dream is a blend of thoughts, concerns, interactions, and activities that you experience in your waking life. While your conscious mind sleeps, images appear, memories are stored, emotions are processed, connections are made, and insights emerge. In an ordinary dream, you are the actor and the observer, the creator and the critic. You are central to the dream even though your conscious mind cannot control the content of the dream or predict what happens next. Ordinary dreams can mimic day-to-day occurrences, or they can be fantastical. Though your brain is highly active, your conscious mind, while asleep, cannot decipher which images are essential or nonessential.

You may incubate and influence an ordinary dream, but you cannot stop yourself from dreaming at will. Dreams occur whether you want them to or not. Whether you remember them or not, they come multiple times each night. They can reoccur, but many are forgotten, particularly the ones that occur earlier in the night. They can be a series of seemingly unrelated images, or they can seem perfectly orchestrated. In an ordinary dream, you do not realize you are dreaming until you awaken. However, an ordinary dream can transform into a lucid dream as soon as you suspect that you are dreaming.

Date: January 20, 2021
Day of Week: Wednesday
Time: 5:46 a.m.

TITLE OF DREAM/THEME: *Being Carried over Unknown Seas*

PEOPLE/PLACES/THINGS: *My home, the sky, military jets, helicopter, unknown village*

FEELINGS/EMOTIONS: *(During or after waking) Ease, no expectations, curiosity*

COLORS: *Blue, bronze*

SYMBOLS: *Jets, helicopter, time on the clock 8:07 a.m., sky, sea*

DETAILS: *I am in my kitchen tidying up before getting ready to go to my office. I look at the clock and it reads 8:07 a.m. I go upstairs, intending to take a shower, but notice that the bathroom is arranged differently. The tub is positioned directly in front of the bathroom door. I then realize that I'm dreaming. I begin to feel the vibrating sensation that typically precedes a lucid dream. I observe what happens next.*

I am being carried through the sky by an unknown force. Military jets fly by, but I feel no fear. They seem to be unaware of my presence. I look at the sea below and begin to descend toward the water. Still no fear—just curiosity. I am now hovering just above the ocean when a bronze-colored helicopter appears and accompanies me. I recognize that I am traveling east at the same pace as the helicopter. We arrive together at an unfamiliar village. The clothing worn by the villagers reminds me of earlier periods in history. Everyone goes about their day. They too are unaware of my presence. I wake up.

INSPIRED ACTION STEPS/CHANGES/DECISIONS: *I allow myself to be carried during times of uncertainty. I embrace unfamiliar paths that lead to new discoveries. I remain curious about the significance of traveling east. Perhaps I am meant to explore and learn more about the cardinal directions of north, south, east, and west.*

CARDINAL DIRECTIONS IN DREAMS

Our ancestors grew to understand the earth's cycles by observing the sun, moon, and other celestial bodies. The cardinal directions in particular were derived from the movement and position of the sun. The word *east* comes from the Greek *auōs,* which means "dawn," while the origin of *north* is believed to be *ner-,* the translation of the earliest Indo-European word for "left." When facing the rising sun, north is the direction to the left of the sun. *West* is derived from another Indo-European word, *wespero-,* which meant "evening," and *south* was translated from *sāwel,* a word that simply meant "the sun."

North

When the direction of north is highlighted in a dream by the location of an object, an animal, or by your position, it often symbolizes greater understanding of deeper mysteries. It represents acquired knowledge over time, through endurance and patience.

East

East is the direction of the rising sun. Traveling toward the east in a dream could be interpreted as approaching greater clarity. A new dawn brings the light of awareness, helping you to see more clearly what is before you.

West

West is the direction of the setting sun, heralding darkness. Darkness is not simply the absence of light. It is a time of introspection, a time of completion, or a time of vital rest.

South

The south is where the sun is hottest. When highlighted by your dreaming mind, the direction of south is a symbol of growth and renewal. This could signal that you are growing toward your highest potential.

NUMBERS IN DREAMS

Numbers can appear in dreams on a clock, mailbox, house, phone screen or license plate, in conversation, or simply written down. If a number is highlighted in a dream, chances are it is significant. Pay attention to how this number appears in waking life. If it was spoken to you by someone you know, ask that person what that number could signify to them. Share that you had a dream in which they mentioned the number and you are curious about its significance. Recently I dreamed of being at an arcade with a friend who said to me in the dream, "I have 45 tickets left." Incidentally, I had not been to an arcade in many years. When I asked my friend what the number 45 signifies to him, the first thing he thought of was the vinyl 45 records that were created in the 1940s. His thought was that my dream was pointing toward a song. As it turns out, he was right. Driving home from my office the following day, what spontaneously entered my mind was Psalm 45, a sacred song found in a collection of hymns in the Old Testament of the Hebrew Bible.

Psalm 45 – NIV: My heart is stirred by a noble theme as I recite my verses for the king; my tongue is the pen of a skillful writer.

COLORS IN DREAMS

Like other dream symbolism, it is essential to determine what colors signify to you, personally, culturally, or otherwise. What feelings surface when you think of gray clouds, blue skies, dark nights, pink flowers, white candles? Red is a vibrant color that is often associated with passion or anger. In some cultures, early Egyptians associated the color red with blood, life, and the divine, believing it offered protection, while West Africans associate red with sacrifice and mourning. What if you dreamed of a purple butterfly fluttering above a female relative lying in a hospital bed? Purple has been associated with heightened intuition and healing abilities, as well as royalty. Green is another color that is associated with healing. As plants are green, the color can also symbolize growth and transformation.

INSIGHTFUL DREAMS

An ordinary dream might come simply to remind you to pay attention and notice the wonders of this waking life. With the busyness of modern living, it is all too easy to become disenchanted with the natural beauty that surrounds you. The sense of awe that you experience in a dream or upon waking is the voice of your inner being nudging you to remember.

Date: June 3, 2016
Day of Week: Friday
Time: 3:11 a.m.

TITLE OF DREAM/THEME: *Remember to Look to the Night Sky*

PEOPLE/PLACES/THINGS: *Unfamiliar cottage, rosebush with red roses, the night sky*

FEELINGS/EMOTIONS: *(During or after waking) Awe*

COLORS: *Dark night, white, red*

SYMBOLS: *Cottage, smoke, candle, rosebush, sky*

DETAILS: *I am standing on the outside of an unfamiliar cottage. There is a screened porch and smoke is rising from the floor. I look closer and see that the smoke is coming from a white candle. My attention moves to a nearby rosebush with red roses. I approach the rosebush and touch the roses. I realize I can feel the roses though I suspect that I am still asleep and dreaming. It feels so real. I look up at the night sky and I feel a sense of awe. I wake up.*

INSPIRED ACTION STEPS/CHANGES/DECISIONS: *It's been a while since I spent some time looking up at the night sky. I will do so tonight before bed.*

Dreams can also reveal how we are navigating through life. Cars, aircraft, and other vehicles transport us from one place to another. These ordinary dream symbols can represent a dreamer's career decisions, educational goals, or other worthwhile pursuits. Combined with other details of the dream, they can convey how someone is making the transition from one stage of life to another. Are you the driver, the front passenger, or in the back seat? Are you clear about which direction you are heading? Are you traveling to a known or unknown destination? To dream of not being able to find where you parked your car might represent a period of indecision or inaction. To find that your car will not start in a dream might indicate the need to pause and consider your next steps before heading in any direction. To dream of a car crash might signal the need to slow down not just when you're in the driver's seat but also if you are hastily moving about your day from one thing to the next. To dream you are a passenger of a car involved in a crash might have an entirely different meaning, that you are being taken on a ride or journey in life that you don't feel you have control over.

An ordinary dream can prepare you for future events. It can provide an honest mirror, allowing you to see yourself as you really are. It can also give you permission to honor your present limitations. There are times when you might need more preparation, growth, or healing before you are ready to enter a new stage of your life, begin a new career, or commit fully to a long-held dream. All of this can be reflected in a seemingly ordinary dream as in the following example.

Date: February 14, 2015
Day of Week: Saturday
Time: 3:13 a.m.

TITLE OF DREAM/THEME: *An Empty Driver's Seat*

PEOPLE/PLACES/THINGS: *Along a dark road, unknown male*

FEELINGS/EMOTIONS: *(During or after waking) Curiosity*

COLORS: *Dark night*

SYMBOLS: *Car, a male presence*

DETAILS: *I am walking along an unfamiliar street. It is dark and I am alone. A car approaches and stops beside me. I look through the front window and notice that there is no one in the driver's seat or passenger seat. In the back seat, there is man who does not look familiar. I am aware that the expectation is for me to get into the driver's seat, but I choose not to. There is no exchange of words. I continue walking in the direction I was headed.*

INSPIRED ACTION STEPS/CHANGES/DECISIONS: *I'm not sure.*

At the time, this dream presented more questions than answers. Was this an invitation to alter my current course? Who was the male presence in the back seat? Had I been subconsciously placing an aspect of myself in the back seat? Was I passing up an opportunity to take greater control of the direction of my life? If so, why did my dreaming mind choose to walk alone in the dark rather than assume the driver's seat?

Many of our dreams invite us to live the mystery of this human experience. At times there is no immediate answer or concrete interpretation. "Not every empty space is meant to be filled" is the message that now emerges when I reflect on this dream from years ago. Empty spaces are necessary to the greater order of things, just as weaknesses and imperfections are essential components of wholeness. Our dreams, no matter how ordinary they might seem, are often leading us to wholeness. For me, that empty driver's seat represented something I was working toward but not yet ready to claim. As for walking alone in the dark, I believe in benevolent unseen forces that walk beside all of us.

BIG DREAMS

The phrase "Big Dreams" was coined by Carl Jung to describe the most vivid, emotionally intense, and transformative dream experiences. Unlike ordinary dreams that might vanish in an instant, big dreams are forever etched in the dreamer's memory. The intensity and vivid imagery of these dreams allow for effortless recall, even if they occurred in early childhood. These dreams might contain no parallels to the dreamer's current waking life. Still, they are often significant and lead to remarkable discoveries and life-changing insights. Some are found to be prophetic, accurately predicting a future event.

Children's Dreams

Big dreams have been found to be most common in children and teenagers. Dream researchers report that children begin having vivid dreams around the age of two. As their imagination begins to develop between the ages of five and nine, their dreams tend to become longer and more complex, and their ability for dream recall increases.[2] Though nightmares are common, children can have other memorable dreams because they are still in touch with the sacred aspect of their innermost being. Even if the child doesn't express or document those dreams, the dreams remain alive.

Faith's Big Dream

Faith, now in her 40s, still remembers a dream she had when she was in kindergarten. She dreamed that she was floating inside what looked like a bubble, and there was another little girl that looked exactly like her. The little girl told her that she was her sister. While in her kindergarten class one day, Faith drew a picture of a bubble with her version of two little girls inside. She does not remember telling anyone about the dream at that time. Years later when she came across the drawing, she immediately remembered the dream. After a few days of thinking about it, she decided to ask her mom, "Did I have a twin sister who died?" Faith told her mom about the dream she had when she was five and showed her the drawing. Her mom admitted that Faith was a twin and that the other baby, another girl, had died in utero. Psychologists confirm that even in utero losses can be felt by the surviving twin. Though Faith had younger siblings, she often felt that something was missing. She was unable to put her feelings into words. Her dreaming mind, however, gave her an image that helped to validate how she felt. It also gave her mom an opportunity to share about a loss that had continued to weigh heavily on her. Knowing that the twin connection transcended death brought them both a sense of comfort.

Hope's Big Dream

When I was 15, I dreamed of being on a hot-air balloon ride. I have never been in a hot-air balloon, but it seemed real. I could feel the air around me, and I could see other balloons with passengers in front of me. Then I saw two hot-air balloons collide. One balloon struck the underside of the balloon that was right above it. The lower balloon began to fall quickly toward the ground. I could see the faces of the people inside. I felt such a sense of horror that I woke up. I vowed never to get into a hot-air balloon.

The images were so vivid that Hope was unable to forget this dream. About a week later, she overheard two women talking about a hot-air balloon accident. The women were from Australia. She recalls her heart racing as she listened to the details. Thirteen people were on board. Tragically, they all died. Hope did not have a personal connection to any of the victims. She was convinced that the details of the accident were the same as her dream. She was moved to pray for the victims. "That was the first time I remember praying for people I didn't know. I think I was just meant to pray for them," she said. "Why else would I have had this dream?"

Hope could not remember anything that could possibly have triggered this dream. Even now she feels that this dream was beyond coincidence. She considers herself an "intercessor," someone who intervenes for another person through prayer. Whenever she dreams of any sort of accident, she says a prayer for anyone who might be involved. She sends a quiet blessing whenever she hears an ambulance go by.

Ancient Indigenous cultures from all corners of the world, including those in Africa, North and South America, and Australia, innately knew that big dreams held wisdom and guidance to aid the wider community. Big dreams offered protection from danger, natural disaster, and famine, as well as healing from disease. Shamans and other spiritual healers with the ability to tap into the mystical became trusted voices to interpret these dreams in a way that benefited the entire community. Cultures that revered these gifts gave rise to other dreamers who made extraordinary contributions to humanity. For instance, American abolitionist Harriet Tubman relied on her dreams and visions to guide other slaves to freedom. Historian Erica Armstrong Dunbar cites a head injury as the cause of Tubman's visionary dreams. Nevertheless, because of her dreams, she knew exactly which trails to follow to avoid capture.

In more recent times, numerous people have reported dreams relevant to world events. For example, based on research conducted by members of the International Association for the Study of Dreams (IASD), there were many dreams featuring plane crashes and building collapses in the weeks preceding September 11.[3] While quantum physics explains our connectedness beyond the physical, science cannot yet explain how these phenomena and other patterns of dreaming happen. Yet we cannot outright deny what cannot be fully understood. We can, however, continue to share our experiences and believe in the mystery.

Beyond survival, various sacred texts relate big dreams that have inspired many generations. Big dreams provide hope, healing, and transformation. They might feature a mystical encounter with a divine presence or other spiritual being. They can speak to the wisdom of nature. They can speak to our ancestry.

ANCESTRAL DREAMS

Carl Jung believed that deeply rooted beliefs, fears, and other behavioral patterns were inherited from our ancestors. He proposed the concept of the "collective unconscious" to explain our shared ancestral experience. This means that even if someone has never experienced a near drowning, that person could still be terrified to go near the sea. Being fearful of bodies of water, also known as thalassophobia, could be an inherited trait, confirms Kendra Cherry, a psychosocial rehabilitation specialist.[4] Based on research by Erik K. Loken and his colleagues at the Virginia Institute for Psychiatric and Behavioral Genetics, this is also true of phobias related to being in crowds, as well as to bridges, snakes, spiders, and other phobias that are not rooted in a personal experience.[5] There is compelling evidence of "transgenerational epigenetic inheritance," where DNA is encoded with memories of traumatic events, adaptations, and instincts that are passed on to subsequent generations. I now believe that these ancestral memories can also manifest in our dreams.

Date: May 10, 2015
Day of Week: Sunday
Time: 3:13 a.m.

TITLE OF DREAM/THEME: *Being Washed Ashore*

PEOPLE/PLACES/THINGS: *The sand, my hands, coconut trees, the sky*

FEELINGS/EMOTIONS: *(During or after waking) Amazement, disbelief*

COLORS: *White, blue, green*

SYMBOLS: *Sky, sandy beach, coconut trees*

DETAILS: *I lift my head up off the sand. It feels as though I've just been washed ashore. The sky is clear blue. The trees are tall, bearing coconuts. I feel a sense of awe at this beautiful scene before me. The colors are vibrant, and it all seems so real. I stare at the palms of my hands. These are my hands. I am aware that this is all a dream. I hear myself say, "There's no way I could be here." I wake up.*

INSPIRED ACTION STEPS/CHANGES/DECISIONS: *Allow this dream to reveal itself to me.*

Then, I had this dream:

May 11, 2015: *I am on a beach with tall coconut trees. I notice a ship up ahead on the beach. It is damaged, torn apart. It looks like an old shipwreck. I walk toward the shipwreck. I wake up.*

Then about two weeks later:

May 23, 2015: *I am walking on the beach. I notice a shiny object lying on the sand. As I get closer, I see it's a mirror. I pick up the mirror and look into it. Instead of*

*seeing my own face, I see the face of another woman. I
close my eyes and I look again. I see another face. Each
time I look, the face in the mirror changes to that of
another woman I do not recognize.*

I decided to share this series of dreams with a friend.
As I spoke of the faces in the mirror, it felt as though I knew
these women, although I did not recognize any of them.
It occurred to me that my dreaming mind could be showing me pieces of my ancestral story, and that I was seeing
all the women who came before me, all the women who
made up pieces of me. Soon after, I also did a search of my
maiden name, Webster, and shipwrecks in Anguilla. This
is when I found a book by Michael Aceto and Jeffrey P. Williams that told of a shipwreck that brought three brothers
with the surname Webster to the island of Anguilla. Imagine my surprise when I first read these words:

> The ship was the English brigantine *Antelope*
> which had left Grenada for England in 1771 (Ber-
> glund 1995:5). Ethnohistorical accounts state that
> there were only three survivors of the shipwreck—
> all brothers sharing the surname Webster. They are
> thought to have made their way to the main island
> of Anguilla shortly after the wreck, in search of a
> source of fresh water.[6]

WORKING WITH BIG DREAMS

The key to working with a big dream is to recognize
that it could be weeks, months, or even decades before
the full message of the dream is revealed. These dreams
extend beyond personal experience and can have a last-
ing impact. Because of their vivid nature, big dreams can

cause us to question reality. They can cause us to doubt ourselves. Carl Jung had a series of dreams preceding World War I that caused him to doubt his mental faculties. It was only after the war began that he recognized his dreams were not indicative of psychosis—rather, they seemed to symbolize the horrors that would befall Europe in 1914.

Try the following steps to work with your own big dreams.

1. First, recognize that this dream chose to come to you at a particular time in your life. Even when you incubate elements of the dream, you cannot control all the details that appear.

2. As you record the dream, invite it to reveal itself to you. This can be done by writing, painting, or drawing whatever comes to mind after you have recorded the dream, or by observing how the dream continues to unfold. Release any expectations of how and when the entire message of the dream will be revealed.

3. Speak the dream aloud to hear its immediate message more clearly. If appropriate, share the dream with someone who appeared in the dream. Chances are, it holds meaning for them too. At the very least, they might be able to contribute to your understanding of the dream.

4. Recognize that big dreams evolve as you do. Continue to record the evolution of these dreams in your journal. What other insights

were realized days, weeks, months, or years later? Be sure to include the date whenever you update a previous journal entry.

5. Revisit big dreams during times of uncertainty and upheaval to see what wisdom they might hold. Remember that big dreams typically serve a purpose beyond your personal life and current circumstances.

DREAM VISUALIZATION PRACTICE: A TREASURED MESSAGE FROM THE DEEP

Dreamscape: On a sandy beach at sunrise.

Objective(s): To experience the revitalizing energy of the morning sun with your inner vision. To contemplate a message from your deeper wisdom.

Visualization: Begin by finding a comfortable position. Allow your body to gently relax.

With your eyes closed, bring your awareness to your heart center.
Breathe in deeply. Breathe out slowly. (Repeat three times.)

With every inhale, allow your entire body to relax further and further. With every exhale, feel a greater sense of ease and surrender. Now, using your imagination, place yourself on a sandy beach near the sea. It is early morning, just before sunrise. See yourself either sitting near the sea or walking along the beach.

Know that you are safe, that you are supported, that you are protected. Feel the air around you, a gentle ocean breeze. Notice how it feels against your skin.

With your inner eyes, look to the horizon. Imagine the fiery sun as it begins to rise, ushering in a brand-new day. Notice the shifting clouds and the vibrant colors that begin to paint the morning sky.

Feel the life force of this morning light, the first light of another day. Feel this enlivening energy as it courses throughout your entire body, encapsulating every cell. Feel how this light invigorates every aspect of you.

Now, hear the ocean waves caressing the shore as you notice something floating in the water right at the shoreline.

Imagine yourself walking over to retrieve what turns out to be a bottle with a folded message inside.

How far has this message traveled to reach you at this time, on this day?

Imagine opening the bottle to read a message that is meaningful to you.

What might this message read?

I offer you these words . . .

As you navigate life's uncertain seas, live and act from your deepest self. Look to the horizon to become more grounded. Allow your inner compass to guide you whenever you feel adrift or lose sight of the shore. Trust that every voyage taken will lead you to uncover more of who you are.

Embodiment: Gently allow yourself to return to the present moment and to your breath. Spend some time with the message or messages that you received. Set the intention to allow yourself to be guided, especially when you feel adrift.

Chapter 8

DREAM VISITORS, KNOWN AND UNKNOWN

My grandmother transitioned into the realm of Spirit on May 31, 1999. I had been to Anguilla that previous March and spent a week with her. I did not allow myself to think that this would be our last time together though she was ill. In the two months since my visit, I had moved into a new apartment in Upstate New York, graduated from chiropractic school, and was about to start a new position at the college's chiropractic clinic. Just as I was moving into another stage of life, so was she. Moments before I received the call, a green moth appeared at the glass sliding door on the deck of my apartment. It looked as though it was glowing, which I later learned is a feature of a luna moth. Mesmerized by its glow, I was a bit startled when the phone rang. It was my mom calling to say that my grandmother had just died. I immediately looked to the glass sliding door; the glowing moth was gone.

Nearly four years passed before my grandmother first appeared in my dreams. When she did, she looked exactly as she did in her later years. She would often smile without saying anything. I would wake up feeling a deep sense of peace. I often dreamed of her back in her home in Anguilla. Other times, the dream occurred in places we had never experienced together in this life, such as my office or at my home. Once in a dream I had given her a glass of water. "You're not supposed to give anything to the deceased," I was later told by a family member. However, the glass of water reminded me of the week I spent caring for her— assisting her with her baths, her meals, and massaging her feet—just as she cared for me in my earlier years. I now believe that the glass of water was my inner psyche's way of inviting her to continue to accompany me in this life.

In November 2007, I dreamed I walked into my bedroom and she was sitting on my bed, holding a baby girl. "What are you doing here?" I asked. After I reminded her that she could not possibly be here because she had died, she disappeared. I was 11 weeks pregnant at the time. This is what I wrote the next morning.

> November 23, 2007: *I am hoping that this dream holds no meaning. I love you already, baby. I want so much for you to enter this world and be a part of our family. It doesn't matter whether you are a boy or a girl, just that you are.*

Two weeks later, I miscarried the pregnancy at 13 weeks gestation. It was later confirmed that had I carried this pregnancy to term, we would have had another girl.

VISITATIONS

If you have ever been visited by a loved one in a dream, you would immediately know it. Visitation dreams engage all of your senses, causing you to feel as though your loved one is present. But unlike a lucid dream, you are unaware that you are dreaming. As you awaken, it could take a moment to reorient yourself and realize that it had been a dream. Typically, there is a deep feeling of peace after a visitation dream. There is a strong sense that your loved one is no longer suffering. If the person had been ill, they might appear more vibrant or as they did prior to illness. They could appear younger. Even if you are observing them at a distance, you know without a doubt that it is them.

Though visitation dreams can come soon after a loss to help process feelings of sadness and other emotions of grief, they could occur at any time. A loved one could come in a dream to say good-bye even before their final breath leaves the body, helping you to see that your connection transcends the physical. Visitation dreams can also be incubated, or they can occur spontaneously. There can be one clear message or multiple messages in a visitation dream that can evolve with time. The following shares a visitation dream that evolved over a course of a week.

September 20, 2020: *One week ago, I shared on my public Facebook page about a dream of my grandfather who passed on about 30 years ago. In that dream, my grandfather accompanied me into a jewelry store and stood beside me as I selected an opalescent ring in the shape of a lamb. He was expressionless and remained silent.*

My interpretation was that the ring signified a commitment and the lamb symbolized gentleness. My grandfather was a gentle and affirming presence and I saw this dream as a reminder to remain true to my gentleness, even though the loudest, most controversial voices are often most easily heard.

Still, I remained curious about the fact that this visitation occurred specifically in a jewelry store when I am not inclined to purchase jewelry. My mom, however, has worked at the same jewelry store since I was a child. Yesterday morning, that store was robbed at gunpoint. While traumatizing, all lives were spared. I spoke to my mom again this morning, and she is in good health and well supported.

Surprisingly, I did not feel a sense of panic when I answered the call and listened as my sister recounted what had occurred. Almost immediately, I was able to recognize the grace that had been present that morning. I believe that somehow my grandfather made certain that my mom would be okay. Just hours before, I had also recited these prayerful words by Caroline Myss, "Shine your grace of love and healing upon those I love and all humanity—the souls I share this journey of life with each day."[1]

THE COLLECTIVE UNCONSCIOUS

In the collective unconscious, we are not merely strangers. This became clear through a connection with a young woman named Krista who passed away unexpectedly in August 2011. I did not know Krista, or any member of her family, before this time. I learned of her family's tragic loss through a social media post by a mutual friend. From the comments, I gathered that she was a generous soul, known for her smile, that she was quick to offer a kind word and sparked much laughter with her sense of humor. "Larger than life" is how many described her personality. While we can never fully understand the pain of another, in her I saw aspects of myself: someone adept at wearing a smile to silently mask the hurt inside. The pain of recurring loss had dismantled my facade. For her, she was not ready to let anyone else in. Though she was loved and adored by many, she succumbed to the loneliness of pain.

Seven months later, at a local library, her mom unexpectedly showed up at my first book signing. I shared how learning about her daughter helped me to see myself more clearly. We talked about how some of us become masterful at minimizing and hiding even though we know how much we are loved. No one else notices because we do not wish to be noticed, or we present only what we want others to see. This is our mechanism for survival. We choose our words carefully and may use humor or shyness as a shield. We know we are loved, but we must find a way to love and accept ourselves enough to recognize that some burdens are too heavy to carry alone. Only when we learn to truly value ourselves do we realize that asking for help is not a sign of weakness or failure.

Krista first appeared in an early-morning dream in May 2012. I could hear my daughter calling to me, but I was drifting back to sleep when an image of Krista's face spontaneously came to mind, startling me awake. I immediately got out of bed, just moments before my daughter fainted and I was there to catch her. I cannot say with absolute certainty what caused Krista's face to appear in that moment since I could not recall any recent thoughts of her. Yet some aspect of me knew exactly what it would take to wake me fully.

In other dreams, Krista is often at a large family gathering with members of her family, some of them I recognize. Other times she appears sitting on a park bench writing in her journal. One morning I woke up remembering a fragment of a paragraph she had written. It read, "to be whole . . ." Those were the only words I could recall. As I sat with my own journal, these words emerged from within me:

> *To be whole does not mean that we were never broken. To be whole means that we embrace all parts of ourselves rather than hide, deny, or disguise. We acknowledge the hurt we feel, and we acknowledge the hurt we may have caused. To be whole means that we recover what is essential within us. We then bring this essence to every relationship, friendship, or romance. We allow others to see the real us, rather than varying personas, dependent on roles and expectations. To be whole means that sometimes we must protect ourselves from those who are choosing an alternate path. They too will find wholeness in their own time and in their own way. Still, we must recognize our need for others to accompany us on this winding road.*

I cannot say that these were Krista's words, but I sense that her mission is linked with mine. She too was an avid writer and kept journals since childhood. She was a poet who cared deeply about the world around her and the people in it. She also adored and cared for children and had hoped to mother her own, one of her sisters had shared. It feels as though she is finally doing so.

When Carl Jung spoke of the collective unconscious, he was referring to our shared human experience, beyond personal influences and cultural expressions. His observations consistently revealed that certain instincts, reactions, and behaviors were inherited, not learned. These intrinsic patterns and themes were not only necessary for survival but also the need to live a life of purpose and meaning. Themes of birth and rebirth, pilgrimage and the return, the shadow and its unrealized potential are experienced by everyone, no matter when and where they were born. There are also personified patterns such as the self; the mother; the child; the wise elder; the anima, described as the feminine aspect of a man's psyche; and the animus, the masculine aspect of a woman's psyche. Jung used the term *archetypes* to categorize these patterns that continuously inform and shape our lives as well as our relationships.

It is essential to note that these archetypes serve only as a blueprint and can be expressed in various ways. Consider the mother archetype; mothering is not exclusive to mothers or even to people who have birthed a child. Likewise, fathering is not exclusive to fathers or people who have biologically fathered a child. The mother archetype also represents grandmothers, stepmothers, mothers-in-law, Mother Nature, and other forms of mothering.

These archetypal patterns can manifest positively and negatively. For instance, the shadow is often seen as the rejected parts of ourselves that we wish to avoid and deny. In facing our shadows, we begin to uncover abilities and transformative gifts that may otherwise remain hidden. Most Jungian analysts agree that the shadow is the most obvious path to realizing our full potential.

When an archetype appears in your dream, it is an opportunity to see your life in a larger context, and to realize that you are not alone in your current challenges. The intention is not to overidentify with any one archetype, but to allow it to reveal aspects of yourself that existed in your ancestors and now exist in all others. See the archetype as a member of your spirit team, helping you to live more freely, to change your trajectory if necessary, and to align with greater purpose.

To learn more about why an archetype has appeared to you, try this exercise in your waking life: Sit comfortably and imagine the archetypal image sitting directly in front of you. Using your imagination, allow the archetype to speak. Each archetypal figure will, in its own words, tell you why it has come.

THE GRANDMOTHER IN DREAMS

The grandmother is the one who carried our mothers and our fathers, who dreamed of us and loved us into being. She is the faithful keeper of traditions, of all that is inherently sacred. She is the giver of dreams, the one who endured unimaginable circumstances so that each of us could exist to uncover our soul's dreams. She is the self-assured matriarch who commands respect not just for herself but also for her children and all her grandchildren. She is the unitive stitch in the tapestry of interconnection. She is the nurturer. She tends, she comforts, she affirms. There is power in her faith, her hope, and her immeasurable love.

The grandmother comes to remind you that you were encoded from the beginning of time with everything needed to transcend your current circumstances. All that existed within her continues to exist within you. Feel the warmth of her embrace. Receive from her strength. Receive from her wisdom. Receive from her love. Live with the certitude that you are nurtured and guided from within.

THE GRANDFATHER IN DREAMS

The grandfather is the provider, the encourager. He keeps a watchful eye, ensuring your safety. He provides structure and guidelines, tools and resources, and mentors when you require guidance for the journey ahead. He then takes a step back so that you may find your own way. Though the father can be fiercely protective, the wise grandfather alerts you to approaching danger and guides you out of harm's way. He compels you to take a course of action, though he watches from a distance, giving his nod of approval. Sometimes he comes near and places his hand on your head or your shoulders.

The grandfather comes to bolster your confidence. He encourages forward movement in a direction that leads to personal fulfillment. He reminds you that you are self-sufficient. Receive from his strength. Receive from his wisdom. Receive from his love. Know that you are safe and supported and always held in his heart.

WISE ELDER IN DREAMS

The wise elder is an adviser with a representation of many voices, communicating in a language that is most easily understood by you. The wise elder is a connector, connecting the past, the present, the future, and all beings. Theirs is not a face you may recognize, but it appears in a form that is comforting to you. The wise elder knows all that you are, your strengths, your weaknesses, and your hidden potential.

The wise elder comes to offer guidance and wisdom at times of great transition for the good of all beings, past, present, and future. The wise elder reminds you that you are accompanied by unseen benevolent forces. Let their strength be your strength. Let their wisdom invoke your deepest wisdom.

THE ANIMA/ANIMUS IN DREAMS

In Latin, *anima* means "soul" and *animus* means "spirit." The anima/animus represents balance and wholeness. Anima is the feminine aspect in males, while animus is the male aspect in females. These aspects offer insight into your complex nature and all that is contained in this human experience. They might wear a face of someone you know so that you might more readily identify the areas in your life where attention is needed, or they could be a mysterious stranger sitting in the back seat of a car with no driver, inviting you to examine your unrealized potential.

The anima/animus comes to provide healing rather than to blame, belittle, or criticize. The anima/animus reminds you that you are not the first nor the last to experience feelings of unworthiness, regret, or envy. They teach that balance replenishes, while imbalance depletes your resources. They are a bridge to truer expression, harmonious balance, and wholeness—rather than perfection.

UNKNOWN DREAM FIGURES

Unknown dream figures allow us to see beyond known personalities and bring into focus our shared humanity.

They highlight our inherent need for community and connection, while honoring our individuality in the process. Each prominent dream character holds a unique aspect to be explored and contributes to the themes presented in the dream.

Date: April 2, 2021
Day of Week: Friday
Time: 5:38 a.m.

TITLE OF DREAM/THEME: *The Young Boy, the Breadmaker, and the Grandmotherly Figure*

PEOPLE/PLACES/THINGS: *Unknown home, unknown "relatives," unfamiliar bread machine*

FEELINGS/EMOTIONS: *(During or after waking) Welcomed, hopeful, joyful*

COLORS: *I can't recall.*

SYMBOLS: *Family, bread*

DETAILS: *I am at a gathering held in an unfamiliar home. The home has multiple levels. There are women and men and children of all ages, almost like a family reunion. But there is no one I recognize. Everyone seems welcoming. In the kitchen, I watch as a male figure removes freshly baked bread from an unfamiliar bread machine. He offers me a piece. I accept. As I get ready to leave, there are many warm embraces, encouraging words, and well wishes. A young boy about the age of 10 says to me, "If you ever need anything, let me know." As I exit the building, I look back and there is a grandmotherly figure standing on a second-floor balcony looking down at me. Her hands are held over her heart, one hand on top of the other. I stare at her. Her gaze appears to be fixed on me.*

INSPIRED ACTION STEPS/CHANGES/DECISIONS: *To continue to explore this dream*

DREAM EXPLORATION

Though unknown to me, these dream figures brought a warmth and kindness that allowed me to feel cared for and hopeful. Their embraces provided comfort at a time when I missed being in community during the continuing pandemic.

When I explore the image of the little boy, I see him as an aspect of my innermost self. His words serve to continuously remind me that I can ask for and receive guidance from my inner being. His essence reminds me to keep my heart open to life and to others. We often forget about our 10-year-old self, the one who was curious about everything the world had to offer, programmed for survival no matter the experience. Or maybe it's not that we forget but that the bright-eyed aspect of our soul gets buried under years of heavy burdens that become too much to bear.

The bread machine is a curious image. It looked like a metal contraption, more complicated than any bread machine I have ever seen. I imagine this was my psyche's way of highlighting the bread. The phrase, "the bread of life" comes to mind, symbolizing an offer of deeper nourishment.

Then, there is grandmother or wise elder with hands over heart. As I allow grandmother's presence to come to life inside me and flow from my pen into my journal, these words emerge: "Protect your heart," Grandmother says. "Do not carry the weight of other people's opinions day after day."

While we are wired to be in community and to seek a sense of belonging, we must also honor the callings of our own heart. The beauty and mystery of this existence is that there is not just one way of being in this world.

HOW TO EXPLORE DREAM VISITATIONS

1. Record the details of the dream and give it a title.

2. Relate the dream to your current waking life experience. Is this visitation to provide comfort, hope, connection, protection, or does it have another purpose?

3. Invite each dream figure, known or unknown, to be present to you in your waking state and speak through your intuitive sense.

4. Explore curious images. What is the dream purposefully highlighting?

5. Does this dream connect to any other recent dreams?

6. Consider how you are being invited to keep the memory of your loved one alive. How are they encouraging you to live your life more fully?

7. Return to the dream whenever other insights arise.

DREAM VISUALIZATION PRACTICE: GATHERING AT THE TABLE WITH YOUR SPIRIT TEAM

This practice is inspired in part by a tradition of the Dagara people in West Africa. Shamans would communicate with the life force of the fetus while still in its mother's womb to discover why it was coming into the world at that particular time and what gifts it might hold for the community. A council of elders would identify the chosen purpose of this new life. Once the child was born, it is believed that the invisible world of Spirit and the ever-present ancestors continued to provide guidance through intuition and dreams.

Dreamscape: A stone cottage in a semirural location

Objective(s): To introduce you to your current Spirit team

Visualization: I invite you to begin by placing your hands on, above, or below your heart, whatever feels comfortable for you.

Breathe deeply and observe your body's response to the breath of life that courses through you, the same breath that was breathed by your ancestors and mine.

Imagine that you have received an invitation from the invisible realm to meet with your Spirit team, a group of guides and guardians that have been assigned to you from before you were born. The meeting is to remind you of why you are here in this life, at this time in history. You will also be able to share concerns, ask for guidance, and make requests. This meeting is to take place in your dreams.

Imagine falling asleep and in your dream, you arrive at a stone cottage. There is a handwritten note on the wooden door that reads, "Come in. You are welcome here."

You are the first to arrive. Inside, you notice that the walls are unfinished, and that there is a pitched roof with wooden beams. In the center of the room is a vintage table and chairs with assigned seating.

You take your seat and await the arrival of your Spirit team. What sensations do you feel in your body as you anticipate their arrival?

Do you hear a song playing in the background? What scents dance in the air?

It is now time to meet your Spirit team.

One by one, they appear before you. Who are they? A loved one in Spirit? A teacher or mentor? A favorite writer or musician? Ancestors? Angels? Divine beings?

They each come over to greet you before taking their assigned seat. Feel each loving embrace, how much you are loved and supported.

After all beings are seated, you are invited to bring whatever concerns you have to the table. Are you seeking healing? Greater connection? A sense of purpose? Speak freely. There is no judgment here, only unconditional love.

What insights or guidance do you receive? Allow this guidance to arise from the deepest part of you.

I offer you this message . . .

You originated from love, declared sacred before you were fully formed. You were chosen for a purpose only you can fulfill through connections only you can make. You are here to expand, to seek what makes you come alive, to transform your greatest fear, to give and receive, to be student and teacher, to find balance, to experience wholeness, and to choose how your evolving story will read.

What else would you like to know in this room where the invisible has been made visible?

It is now time to return to the present time and space. No need to say good-bye because this team, though typically unseen, is always available to you. Now that you know who walks beside you, know that you do not have to carry the burdens of this lifetime alone.

Embodiment: How will your story read? Take some time to consider what truly makes you come alive. What is your greatest fear? What gifts do you hold that might benefit your immediate community? What would you like to give more of, and what would you like to receive more of? Return to this practice whenever you need to be reminded that you are never alone, and that your life has purpose simply because you exist.

Chapter 9

ENGAGING
WITH ANIMAL
ARCHETYPES

There is a Native American legend in which the Creator of all that is gathers with the animals to discuss humans.

"I want to hide something from humans until they are ready," says the Creator. "It is the realization that they create their own reality."

The eagle is first to offer a solution. "Give it to me. I can fly it to the moon," the eagle offers.

"No," the Creator says. "One day soon, they will fly to the moon and find it before many are fully ready."

"I can hide it at the bottom of the sea," says the salmon.

"No, some will go there, too, but they may not recognize that the gift is for all, not just a chosen few."

"What if I bury it deep within the great plains?" the buffalo asks.

"They will dig into the earth and find it, but compare it to other buried treasures," the Creator responds.

147

Then Grandmother Mole, who has no physical eyes, says, "Put it inside them. That will be the last place they will look."

And the Creator says, "It is done."

Dreams guide us inward, allowing us to see the nature of reality. Not only do they enable us to see ourselves more clearly, but they also help us understand the happenings in the world around us. Dreams use what knowledge we already have and then allow us to decide how each symbol relates to our current reality. Even though we all dream, our unique perspectives shape our varying realities and interpretations.

"You cannot rid the world of all its problems," an elder archetype said to me in a dream. He then pointed to a turtle on a log and said, "Turtle has two homes." Looking for additional insight, I shared this dream with friends. "A turtle lives in its shell and in the larger world," one friend offered. "Sometimes we have to retreat into our inner sanctuary and recharge when the world's problems become too overwhelming." Another friend sent an article that revealed that turtles follow the same migratory path to hibernate every year, returning to the exact spot based on tracking and measurements. The article featured a photo of a snapping turtle carrying 18 pounds of soil with grass growing on top. The photo was reminiscent of a Native American myth of the Northeast Woodland tribes about the Great Flood, in which the turtle carries on its back the soil needed to re-create the earth. The symbol of the turtle, then, represents Mother Earth to many Iroquois and Ojibwe people. The Zuni of New Mexico believe that when a child is desired and there is no pregnancy, turtle medicine will boost fertility. To the Taino people of the Caribbean, the turtle is our most ancient ancestor, our fertile mother, a powerful connector because of its ability to live in the sea and on land. In sharing our dreams with others, we receive varying perspectives that can expand our understanding of what the dream wants to reveal to us.

The following section contains five categories of animal archetypes: Messengers of the Night, Messengers of the Air, Messengers of the Waters, Messengers of the Ground, and Pet Messengers. This information includes common traits, archetypal presentations, as well as symbolism, legends, and folklore from various cultures. Our knowledge of the instincts, behaviors, and evolutionary adaptations of animals can provide insight into our own demeanor and adaptive patterns. This knowledge can be greatly influenced by culture and other teachings. An animal might represent a favorable omen in most cultures but symbolize an unwelcome guest in others. You may notice that there is often one well-known interpretation that tends to overshadow other meanings. As the legends and folklore from around the world reveal, all are worthy of being honored.

When it comes to the mystical nature of dreams, the key is to remain open and curious rather than to rely on a single fixed interpretation. Pay close attention to the bodily sensations that arise as you read about each animal. If a legend or story from a particular country or people resonates, consider exploring and learning more about that nation and their traditions. Look to multiple sources for additional information whenever you dream of an animal or have an encounter that feels meaningful. The cautionary message that is shared for each animal was created during meditation, when I invited that animal to speak as I listened deeply.

January 23, 2020: *I am standing alone in my backyard. Through the dark of this night, I notice a bat. Instead of hanging from the tree branch, the bat stands upright, facing the lake. To the right of the bat is a lantern with a brilliant glow. I notice that the lantern and the bat are of similar height and width. The bat's right wing extends as if to hold the lantern. I also observe the lake. There is stillness, no moonlight, just the glow from the lantern.*

MESSENGERS OF THE NIGHT

Bat

Traits: Bats are mammals that emerge from the mother's womb. They are known for their ability to sustain long periods of flight and for their excellent perception, allowing them to find their way through the dark.

Archetypal Image: Though not all bats live in caves, the image of a bat emerging from its cave is representative of emerging consciousness and unrealized potential, of facing our shadows and beginning anew. There is also an association to the trickster archetype derived from the Celtic myth of a destructive enchantress who shape-shifted into a bat.

Indigenous Symbolism: Bat represents the cycle of death and rebirth, most notably in Central American countries such as Guatemala, Belize, Honduras, and northern Costa Rica, as well as in central and southern Mexico. To the Mayan, Aztec, Toltec, and Toluca peoples, bats were sacred.

African Symbolism: Bat is associated with the trickster archetype based on Nigerian folklore and the creation of darkness according to a tale from Sierra Leone.

Eastern Symbolism: Bats are good omens of happiness, longevity, and good fortune in Asian cultures.

Celtic Symbolism: Aside from the trickster archetype, bat is associated with the underworld, and is thus symbolic of Samhain, the Celtic tradition that gave rise to Halloween.

Cautionary Message: Do not deny the darkness. In life, there will often be challenges to face, conflicts to resolve, sad good-byes, and unexpected losses. But alongside that darkness, there will be tender moments, blissful moments, and wondrous moments that make it all worthwhile. Do not lose sight of the light.

Coyote

Traits: Coyotes are known for their intelligence and versality. Though mostly nocturnal, they can be active during the day. They communicate mostly through sound, howling to announce or defend territorial boundaries or to interact with their own pack members.

Archetypal Image: Coyote is a master trickster that allows us to see humanity's foolishness and our own contribution to the "silliness" by either taking life too seriously or not learning from past mistakes.

Indigenous Symbolism: Coyote is seen as playful teacher, mischievous shape-shifter, and powerful magician in Sioux, Navajo, and Cheyenne legends. The Syilx Okanagan and Secwépemc peoples of British Columbia also see the coyote as a trickster.[1]

African Symbolism: Coyote's cousin, the jackal, is most prevalent in African countries. Jackal is also known to be clever and mischievous. In ancient Egypt, jackals were associated with the afterlife.[2]

Eastern Symbolism: The shape-shifting fox, another close relative, is more common in Eastern animal symbolism. In Japan, red fox wards off evil spirits.

Celtic Symbolism: Though uncommon in Celtic regions, coyotes are closely related to dogs and wolves and mostly seen as devoted companions and guides. Their magical nature links them to phantasmagoria, a world of illusion and fantastical events.

Cautionary Message: Be aware of illusions. If someone or something does not seem right, do not betray your intuitive sense. Trust your instincts and ask further questions.

Moth

Traits: Though nocturnal, moths are attracted to the light and fly close to the flame. They navigate by the light of the stars and the moon. Some, like the luna moth, have a life span of one week and their sole purpose is to reproduce. Moths can see the ultraviolet rays that are invisible to human eyes.

Archetypal Image: Moth's attraction to the flame represents the fire archetype. Fire is essential to life, transformation, and the eternal flame of hope. Fire is also destructive if not used responsibly.

Indigenous Symbolism: Similar to the butterfly, moth is sacred, symbolizing growth and transformation. In the South American country of Colombia, the Guajiro people believe that a white moth is the spirit of an ancestor.

African Symbolism: In sub-Saharan Africa, it is believed that certain dark nocturnal moths can embody the soul of an ancestor.[3]

Eastern Symbolism: Moth is believed to carry the soul of the departed. This association came from the abundance of moths found at the Chinese Qingming Festival, where tombstones are swept to honor deceased relatives.

Celtic Symbolism: Other than reference to the death moth, known for its skull-like pattern, moth is not a common symbol in Celtic traditions.

Cautionary Message: As you seek what sparks your passion in life, be aware of overidentifying with your achievements. Your legacy is not just what you leave behind, it is also who you became in the process and the flame you ignited in others along the way.

Opossum

Traits: Known for "playing dead," opossums are the only pouched mammals found in North America. They date back more than 65 million years—when dinosaurs still roamed the earth. Opossums can give birth to as many as 20 babies in one litter, but fewer than half typically survive. Born deaf and blind, a baby opossum must find its way to its mother's pouch.

Archetypal Image: Opossum can be seen as a trickster, displaying wit to outsmart a predator or to avoid confrontation. However, the momentary immobility is an involuntary response to fear. Opossum, then, represents a protective instinct rather than deception.

Indigenous Symbolism: In central Mexico, opossum is symbolic of fertility to the Nahua people. The Mazatec, also indigenous to Mexico, credit opossum with spreading fire to the rest of humanity by taking it from someone who had intended on keeping it to herself.

Cautionary Message: Stand in your truth rather than hide to avoid confrontation. You have the right to say when something does not align with who you are at the present time. You also get to decide how and when to spread light.

Owl

Traits: Owl's eyes are fixed, allowing for incredible focus and depth perception. Owl has superb hearing and can pinpoint the location of sound, even if it cannot see it. Its wings beat silently, allowing it to move about undetected.

Archetypal Image: Owl is the wise elder archetype who understands that wisdom is attained through having experiences rather than gathering information and/or memorizing details. Owl keenly observes and thus sees what is not yet visible. Owl listens deeply to hear beyond what is spoken. It is not easily deceived.

Indigenous Symbolism: Owl represents sacred wisdom and connection to the spirit realm. Healers among the Cherokee people believed that owls provided guidance that enabled them to heal the sick.

African Symbolism: Owl is associated with supernatural and magical influences. To the Bamana people of West Africa, owls were messengers of sad news.[4]

Eastern Symbolism: In Japan, owl is used for protection and ensures good fortune.

Celtic Symbolism: Owl's keen sight and ability for silent travel makes it the perfect guide through the underworld.

Cautionary Message: True wisdom looks with eyes of compassion, not judgment. Seek to understand more and judge less.

Panther

Traits: Panthers, jaguars, and leopards are of the same exquisite species. Panthers are known to be versatile and strong, fearless and aggressive. They are skilled climbers, strong swimmers, and can leap more than 15 feet. They are solitary hunters and are often described as ghostly, as they can go unnoticed in the dark of night.

Archetypal Image: Panther is the ruler of its territory, with unmatched skill and strength. Panther is powerful and self-assured. The panther archetype encourages us to come into our power by living with integrity as we embrace the unknown within ourselves and face our deepest fears.

Indigenous Symbolism: Known as *balam* in Mayan, temples were built in honor of panthers and jaguars in Aztec, Mayan, and Inca cultures.[5] Panthers and jaguars symbolized courage, power, and vision.

African Symbolism: More revered than the lion by the South African Zulu people, panther and African leopard symbolized power, courage, and nobility.[6] In West Africa, leopard represents wisdom.

Eastern Symbolism: Panthers and leopards are known as guardians of sacred spaces.

Celtic Symbolism: Panther is the brave warrior spirit.

Cautionary Message: You do not need to walk alone in the darkness. Allow others to accompany you as you face your greatest challenges. There is strength in unity, and to be vulnerable is an act of bravery.

Wolf

Traits: Wolves are swift and formidable creatures, possessing great stamina and able to survive the most challenging climates. They maintain a complex social structure and demonstrate emotional intelligence, maintaining bonds between members of the pack. Though often depicted as wild and as bloodthirsty werewolves, wolves benefit other species by attacking only the frail and injured animals of the herd.

Archetypal Image: Wolf archetype represents our ability to develop strong emotional bonds, and to remain loyal and fiercely protective of family, especially the young and the frail. Wolf embodies our survival instincts as well, to attack when we feel threatened.

Indigenous Symbolism: Wolf empowers us to trust our instincts and move heaven and earth to protect our young. To the Ojibwe people, wolves are guardians of the underworld, responsible for one's journey from the material realm into the spiritual one.[7]

African Symbolism: In African countries, the jackal is more significant than the wolf and is seen mainly as a trickster. Anubis, an early Egyptian deity with a jackal's head, was considered to be a guide to souls in the afterlife.[8]

Eastern Symbolism: The Japanese word for wolf, *ookami*, means "great spirit."

Celtic Symbolism: Wolf is revered for strength and swiftness.

Cautionary Message: Though you have good instincts, pause and do not rush judgments. Be open to new perspectives, particularly when you feel challenged. Recognize that there is always more to learn.

MESSENGERS OF THE AIR

Blue Heron

Traits: Great blue heron is highly adaptable, majestic in flight with a wingspan of about seven feet. It embraces stillness, wading in shallow waters while patiently awaiting its next catch. Great blue heron has excellent night vision.

Archetypal Image: Blue heron is the explorer archetype, gracefully leading us from one path to another. Blue heron invites us to leave ordinary comforts and wade in unfamiliar waters. With its impeccable vision, blue heron allows us to see the perfection of the universe in an imperfect world and to trust our intuitive sense.

Indigenous Symbolism: Blue heron brings good luck to a fisherman who embraces stillness and patience, even if he stands alone. The Lenape people of the Northeastern Woodlands saw great blue heron as a bridge between the water and the sky. Their "Heron Dance" allowed prayers to be sent to the Great Spirit.[9]

African Symbolism: Blue heron represents balance, stability, and adaptability. Heron is revered by the Bantu people of South Africa.

Eastern Symbolism: In Japan, heron is respected for its ability to connect with three of the four elements: air, water, and earth.

Celtic Symbolism: Herons were associated with gods and goddesses, particularly Rhiannon, the goddess of lakes and waters.

Cautionary Message: Embrace stillness, not isolation. Embrace patience, not stagnation.

Blue Jay

Traits: Like wolves, blue jays are known for their intelligence and close family bonds. Blue jays are loud, musical, and can imitate the scream of a red-shouldered hawk. They use their hawk impression to divert predators and scare other birds away from feeders. Blue jays invade other nests and are also known for anting, wiping away an ant's defensive secretions before eating it.

Archetypal Image: Blue jay is another trickster or jester archetype, using cleverness to outwit predators and deceive other birds. Blue jay encourages boldness and ingenuity when it comes to meeting one's needs. It is expressive and reminds us of our need to be heard.

Indigenous Symbolism: Blue jay embodies air, representing mental focus, clarity, and intelligence. In the Chinook Indian Nation, located along the American Northwest Coast, blue jay is considered a hero as well.

Celtic Symbolism: In Celtic mythology, blue jay was associated with the majestic oak trees that were revered for their resilience and strength. Some say that blue jays were the souls of Druids, notable leaders returning to the sacred forest.

Cautionary Message: Use your voice to inspire and affirm and not to demean or disparage anyone, including yourself. Words that divide lead to destruction. Words that unify lead to creative resolutions.

Dove

Traits: Doves do not have peripheral vision, so they can see only what is directly in front of them. Their renowned cooing is a mating call made mostly by male doves. The mourning dove is so named because of its more somber sound. Doves typically travel in pairs.

Archetypal Image: Dove is the archetype of innocence, allowing for hopefulness and sincere optimism. Dove represents our ability to have faith and to love unconditionally.

Indigenous Symbolism: Dove is a messenger of the spirit world, a messenger of love, and is associated with the Aztec goddess Xochiquetzal and also fertility.

African Symbolism: To the Zulu people of South Africa, the green-spotted dove is a symbol of sorrow and stillness.

Eastern Symbolism: In China, dove bestows long life and inner peace. The dove was associated with the goddess of fertility known as Inanna or Ishtar in parts of what is now western Asia.

Celtic Symbolism: Dove is a messenger of love, peace, and harmony.

Cautionary Message: Though innocence is sometimes bliss, deeper awareness and greater understanding allow for greater peace. Instead of ignoring or denying the chaos, seek to restore harmony, first within yourself.

Dragonfly

Traits: Dragonflies have inhabited Earth for more than 300 million years. They are known to have extraordinary vision, close to 360 degrees. While humans see the world in combinations of red, green, and blue, dragonflies see between 11 and 30 primary colors. How is that for perspective?

Archetypal Image: With its iridescent wings, dragonfly represents the powerful magician archetype. It is also a wise sage, having seen many transitions over millions of years. Dragonfly reminds us that nothing is permanent and that change is the nature of life. Dragonfly asks that we embrace every stage of our lives and allow for the magic and wonder of each day.

Indigenous Symbolism: Dragonfly blesses you with life and good health, guiding you through change, healing, and transformation. Dragonfly medicine is practiced by the Hopi and Pueblo tribes of the American Southwest.

Eastern Symbolism: Japan is known as the Island of the Dragonfly. To the samurai, dragonfly brings strength, protection, and swift victory.

Celtic Symbolism: Celtic fairies were inspired by the magical nature of dragonfly.

Cautionary Message: To resist change would be to resist growth, meaning you would miss the magic, adventure, and wonder of life's many moments.

Eagle

Traits: Eagles awaken at sunrise and fly to high altitudes, higher than any other bird. When a bald eagle loses a feather on one side, it loses a matching feather on the other side to balance itself. A female eagle is known to drop twigs from far heights for a potential mate to catch to test his agility and strength. It is believed that this ensures that the male eagle will be able to safely recover an eaglet if ever one should fall.

Archetypal Image: The eagle archetype represents the freedom to soar to great heights and the expansiveness of the world—our balance between what is known and unknown, our connection to the heavens and to the earth.

Indigenous Symbolism: Eagle is connection to Great Spirit, the Creator of all that is. The Choctaw people, native to the American Southeast, would weave eagle feathers into clothing in order to strengthen the connection between the person who wore the clothes and Great Spirit.[10]

African Symbolism: In Zambia, the African fish eagle represents liberty and abundant beauty.

Eastern Symbolism: Eagle symbolizes great strength. In Indonesia, the mythical eagle Garuda is symbolic of creative energy.[11]

Celtic Symbolism: Eagle provides inspiration, vision, and strength.

Cautionary Message: To achieve balance and soar to great heights, you must be willing to let go of certain tasks that weigh you down. There is freedom in knowing what you were made for and when to make use of the talents and skills of others.

Hawk

Traits: Hawks are known for their elaborate courtship dance, their sharp eyesight, and their speed. Intent on catching their prey, some can travel close to 200 miles per hour.

Archetypal Image: Hawk is the hero archetype, revered for its masterful observational skills and keen vision. Hawk reminds us to pay attention to the guidance we receive, allowing us to persevere when faced with obstacles and to embrace sudden transitions with grace.

Indigenous Symbolism: In Lakota Sioux mythology, hawk spirit bestows clear vision. Hawk is messenger of our ancestors who once walked the earth, offering insight and protection.

African Symbolism: According to Credo Mutwa, a celebrated healer in South Africa, if you dream of a hawk, see it as a calling to something greater. Hawk is sacred, initiating you to higher truths.[12]

Eastern Symbolism: Hawk is a noble and talented warrior. In Japan, a hawk feeding its offspring is said to signify rebirth and hope.

Celtic Symbolism: Hawk is a messenger between realms as well as a purveyor of good instincts.

Cautionary Message: Do not allow reactivity to override your otherwise good instincts or cause you to lose your hawkeyed perspective. Take time to honor your emotions. Focus on what matters most as you evaluate all angles before diving into irreversible action.

Hummingbird

Traits: Hummingbirds are attracted to brightly colored tubular flowers and visit hundreds of blooms each day. Studies reveal that hummingbirds have extraordinary recall and can remember flowers they have been to more than a year previously. Though tiny in size, they can be aggressive, even when face-to-face with a larger bird.

Archetypal Image: The hummingbird archetype recognizes the beauty and joy inherent in nature. Hummingbird reminds us to enjoy the sweet, tender moments with those we love, including those who are no longer with us but never forgotten.

Indigenous Symbolism: Hummingbird is a messenger of joy, beauty, and enduring love from the spirit world. The Aztecs saw the hummingbird as "a symbol of strength in life's struggle to elevate consciousness—to follow your dreams."[13]

Cautionary Message: Do not let the tragedies and suffering of the world cause you to give up on the sweet joys of this life. Remember that joy comes in moments and that each new dawn holds the possibility of more joy-filled moments. To remember this, you need only look at the face of a child.

Ladybug

Traits: Ladybugs, also known as ladybirds, are beetles that were revered by early farmers for feeding plentifully on agricultural pests. Ladybugs are named for the Virgin Mary. Their shell and bright coloring offer great protection from predators. Though typically solitary, they can gather in swarms of thousands to reproduce and hibernate. A female ladybug can delay the fertilization of her eggs for up to three months after mating, allowing her offspring a greater chance of survival. Ladybugs appear to be sensitive to environmental changes.

Archetypal Image: Ladybug is another caregiver archetype, keen on providing a service that is beneficial to as many as possible. Ladybug typically works alone. Ladybug's primary concern is the well-being of others.

Indigenous Symbolism: Ladybug's cousin, the water beetle, is a symbol of renewal and humility. There is a Hopi story that tells of how the black beetles produced much-needed rain. There is also a Cherokee creation myth in which a water beetle retrieved soft mud from below the surface waters that became earth.

Eastern Symbolism: In the Chinese adoption community, ladybug brings good news. If caught and released, ladybug will also fly to your true love and whisper your name.

Celtic Symbolism: Ladybug is a symbol of protection.

Cautionary Message: Recognize your need for adequate rest and your sensitivity to the environment around you. Be sure to replenish your energetic reserves. Choose aliveness instead of overwork and allow others to be the answer to your prayers.

Raven

Traits: Ravens are known mostly for their striking black plumage and clever nature. Recent experiments reveal that they are teachable, capable of bartering and delaying instant gratification. Ravens are sure-footed and inquisitive when on the ground and exhibit buoyancy in their ability to somersault while in flight.[14]

Archetypal Image: Raven is the magician archetype, bringing what has been kept hidden into sight. Raven encourages us to see the dark times not as the end of times but as opportunities to rekindle the light. Raven reminds us to do what is within our power to plan for the future, but then surrender to the greater mystery that provides our every need.

Indigenous Symbolism: A portrayer of darkness and mystery, raven is a bearer of magic and light. In the North American Tahltan legends, raven is a heroic guardian spirit.

Eastern Symbolism: Raven is associated with the sun and divine intervention.

Celtic Symbolism: Raven is protector of warriors, companion to seers, and heralder of death and other earthly happenings.

Cautionary Message: Do not be dismayed when faced with uncertainty. While there is power in knowledge and preplanning, there is also power in acceptance and letting go in peaceful surrender.

MESSENGERS OF THE WATERS

Dolphin

Traits: Dolphins are intelligent, playful, and benevolent creatures with great communication skills. They occupy the world's oceans, seas, and some rivers, but their mammalian lungs require them to come to the surface to breathe. Though they have been known to rescue humans, they can become aggressive when stressed or when one of their pod is threatened.

Archetypal Image: Dolphin represents the caregiver archetype, coming to the rescue and guiding others to safety. Dolphin encourages us to be playful and helpful, to come to the surface to take a deep breath and align with our own natural rhythms.

Indigenous Symbolism: Dolphin is the restorer of the "sacred breath of life."[15] The Indigenous people of Brazil believed that dolphins were enchanted beings who would aid shamanic healers in restoring health.

African Symbolism: Dolphin is the ancient guardian and protector.

Eastern Symbolism: Dolphin is the rescuer, and offers protection to those traveling stormy seas.

Celtic Symbolism: Dolphin symbolizes rebirth and reincarnation.

Cautionary Message: Do not succumb to the anguish of stormy seas. Rise to the surface and take one slow breath and then another. Communicate your needs and be receptive to the guidance and support that is available to you.

Fish

Traits: Fish have existed for more than 500 million years. Without vocal cords, fish communicate through vibrating muscles that create sound. Fish rely on their hearing and a sensory system known as the lateral line that runs from their heads to their tails under their scales. This is how they detect sound, motion, and electrical charges in the water. Lateral lines also allow fish to form and maintain their position in schools, which sometimes number in the millions.

Archetypal Image: The fish archetype represents our sense of belonging to something greater than ourselves and to each other. In the school of life, every person has their rightful place. Fish encourages us to use our inherent sensory gifts to find where we are meant to go next.

Indigenous Symbolism: Salmon symbolizes inner knowing. To the Umatilla people and other tribes of the Pacific Northwest, salmon are sacred, "put here by the Creator for our use as part of the cycle of life." As the legend goes, when the Creator decided that people would inhabit Earth, salmon was first to offer its body to feed the people.[16]

African Symbolism: Fish symbolize fertility and abundant creation to the Yoruba people of southwestern Nigeria. In South Africa, their national fish is the galjoen, known for its fighting spirit and ability to endure rough seas.[17]

Eastern Symbolism: Koi fish is a symbol of perseverance and tenacity. In Buddhism, a pair of golden fish represents happiness and freedom.

Celtic Symbolism: Fish represents wisdom and bestows fertility.

Cautionary Message: You were not born into this abundant life simply to repeat patterns, habits, and behaviors. Attune to your unique sense of knowing and you will be guided to fulfill your most sacred assignment in this school of oneness.

Frog

Traits: Frogs are best known for their adaptability; born in water, they are able to live on dry land, in trees, or deep underground. Most frogs have lungs and can breathe through their skin in oxygen-rich waters. They can survive freezing temperatures by slowing their metabolic processes to such an extreme that they appear to be dead, but they are able to essentially thaw out when the temperature rises.

Archetypal Image: Frog is the rebel archetype, often leaping beyond its habitat just because it can. Frog will survive against the odds, even if it means hibernating for quite some time. Frog reminds us to go past our everyday comforts and embrace our sense of adventure without hesitation or regret.

Indigenous Symbolism: Frog represents cleansing waters and the abundance of transformative cycles to the Coast Salish people of the American Northwest. There is a Tsimshian legend in which the Frog represents the connection between Mother Earth and humanity. The Tsimshian people are also indigenous to the Pacific Northwest coast.[18]

African Symbolism: In ancient Egypt, frog symbolized birth, rebirth, and renewal.

Eastern Symbolism: Frog represents naturally flowing prosperity, transformation, and good fortune.

Celtic Symbolism: Frog is associated with magic and transformation, healing and renewal.

Cautionary Message: Do not be a rebel just because you are afraid that others will not accept you as you are. Likewise, do not lose your individuality for the sake of belonging.

Swan

Traits: Despite their large size, swans can paddle swiftly through water and fly at incredible speeds. They can fall asleep while floating or stand on one foot when on land. Known for their gentleness, elegance, and grace, swans can also be protective of each other and of their young. When two swans put their heads together, their necks form a heart, the symbol of love.

Archetypal Image: Swan is the archetype of grace, gliding effortlessly across the surface of open waters or flying in V-shaped formations without colliding, despite their large size. Swan reminds us to rest and surrender to grace rather than struggle to stay afloat.

Traditional Symbolism: Swan is associated with the Great Spirit in the Lakota Sioux culture.

Eastern Symbolism: In Hinduism, the swan represents sacred knowledge and discerning wisdom.

Celtic Symbolism: Swan is mystical and sacred to the ancient bards who were the keepers of tradition in Scotland and Ireland.

Cautionary Message: The journey inward is not just a spiritual one; it is a journey toward seeing your embodiment as a sacred gift. The journey is not meant to be an internal struggle or battle to remain afloat. It is to be in harmony with yourself and with others.

Whale

Traits: Evolutionary data reveals that whales were originally land dwellers with four legs and hooves before they evolved into mammals of the sea. Whales are intelligent creatures and effective communicators. Some baleen whales, like the humpback and blue whales, create predictable patterns of sounds that can be heard from miles away. These whale songs are sung during mating season, feeding periods, or when mourning. Whales have been found to have the capacity to grieve.

Archetypal Image: The whale archetype represents the search for inner strength when circumstances take you to your depths. Whale reminds you to pause, breathe deeply, and listen to the echoes of hope that will guide you to solid ground.

Traditional Symbolism: To the Kānaka Maoli, the Indigenous Hawaiians, whale represents connection between the physical and spiritual realms.[19] It is believed that ancestors take the shape of whales to provide guidance.

African Symbolism: In one Swahili tale, whale teaches humility to a king who desired to feed all the creatures of Earth. It is not up to one person to solve all the world's problems.[20]

Eastern Symbolism: Lord Vishnu, the Hindu deity believed to be protector of Earth, is said to take the form of a whale. In Vietnam,[2] whale is revered and is addressed as Cá Ông or "Lord Fish."[22]

Celtic Symbolism: Whale provides guidance to those at sea.

Cautionary Message: Unlike whale's land-dwelling ancestors, you cannot simply move to another habitat or fall asleep hoping to awaken when all the suffering of the world is gone. You are here to communicate your "heartsongs"[23] and manifest heaven on this extraordinary earth. As the young poet Mattic Stepanek described, "A heartsong is our inner beauty—our sense of why we are here and how we can keep going. We each have a heartsong, rooted in purpose, or our reason for being."

MESSENGERS OF THE GROUND

Ant

Traits: Ants are known for their incredible strength and survivability. They can carry up to 50 times the weight of their own body. Not only can ants be in water and not drown, but they are also believed to have outlived dinosaurs and survived the Ice Age.

Archetypal Image: The ant archetype encourages collaboration, allowing all members of the community to thrive. Ant is deliberate in tasks and delegates when necessary.

Indigenous Symbolism: Ant works patiently to spread the soil across the earth. In central Mexico, Nahua elders tell of how Quetzalcoatl, an Aztec deity, took the form of an ant to bring nourishment and knowledge from the natural world to humans.[24]

African Symbolism: Ant tells of approaching rain or harvest. To the Kabyle people of Algeria in North Africa, ants were a source of wisdom, sharing their knowledge of the natural world.[25]

Eastern Symbolism: Ant is virtuous and dutiful. In India, there is a parable about a Hindu deity named Indra and the ants. The parable served as a lesson in humility and a reminder that there are always cycles of creation and destruction.[26]

Cautionary Message: Do not carry heavy burdens alone. Just because you can does not mean that you must. Use your talents in ways that honor you and where you are best able to serve.

Bear

Traits: Bears are known for their intelligence, excellent memory, and their superior sense of smell, hearing, and sight. Bears are also known for their ability to care deeply about other bears. Mothers fiercely protect their young, and cubs have been found to grieve the loss of their mother for weeks.

Archetypal Image: Bear often represents the mother archetype, protective and attentive to the needs of the most vulnerable. Bear reminds us to spend time in hibernation to transform all that we have experienced into wisdom. Bear encourages us to graciously mentor others as we share all the wisdom we have gathered.

Traditional Symbolism: Bear symbolizes strength, power, and introspection. To the Haida people of British Columbia, bear is known as "Elder Kinsman" and is a welcomed guest.[27]

African Symbolism: Bear is an unwelcome visitor and evokes fear in the Nandi people who inhabit western Kenya, Tanzania, and Uganda. "Chemosit," or "Chimiset," as the mysterious predator commonly known as Nandi bear is called, translates to "evil spirit."[28]

Eastern Symbolism: The panda bear symbolizes harmony and balance.

Celtic Symbolism: Bear represents strength, courage, and protection.

Cautionary Message: As you seek to protect what is yours, be mindful that your reactions do not cause harm to others. Be merciful when mercy is a viable option.

Deer

Traits: Deer are agile social creatures who travel in herds. They are known to be timid and gentle, and generally run to avoid confrontation. However, they stomp, kick, and use their antlers to attack if they are cornered or perceive a threat to their fawn. Male deer shed their antlers once a year.

Archetypal Image: Deer is the archetype of innocence, enjoying the changing landscapes of each season. Deer reminds us to take notice of our surroundings and enjoy the simple pleasures that exist in the present moment. Deer encourages us to embrace the power inherent in gentleness and compassion.

Indigenous Symbolism: Deer is a gentle yet powerful spirit. When the Lenape people, who originally lived in the eastern United States, came across the "Great White Deer," they innately understood the message of this divine being, to respect all life.[29]

African Symbolism: The red deer, or Barbary Stag, native to Africa, is seen as majestic and worthy of protection in the North African countries of Algeria, Morocco, and Tunisia.[30]

Eastern Symbolism: When the Engakuji Temple in eastern Japan opened its doors for the first time, a herd of white deer appeared at this Zen Buddhist temple. Deer are sacred, symbolizing purity, innocence, and harmony.[31]

Celtic Symbolism: Female deer represent gentleness and grace, while stags are protectors. White deer—a result of a rare genetic variation—are otherworldly messengers.

Cautionary Message: Do not let the harsher realities of life steal away your belief in the goodness that still exists. While anger can be righteous, the world desperately needs gentleness and kindness.

Horse

Traits: Horses are known for their incredible strength and endurance, as well as their sensitivity and loyalty to humans. Their ability to sleep while standing is a matter of survival, as it ensures that they can run quickly from predators. Still, they must lie down to enter the deeper stages of sleep, which is necessary for their brain function.

Archetypal Image: Horse is an explorer archetype, and it values freedom. Horse encourages us to explore various terrains and delight in the traveling winds with a sense of adventure. Horse reminds us to be aware, but not be on constant alert; we must also rest when necessary.

Indigenous Symbolism: The horse is a symbol of strength and power, welcoming humans onto its back. To the Lakota and other Great Plains peoples, horses represented greater ease and flow in daily life.

African Symbolism: The Namibian horse is revered for its adaptability and survivability in hostile environments.[32]

Eastern Symbolism: Horse represents integrity and bravery. The *chollima*, or *qianlima*, which means "thousand-mile horse," is legendary in East Asian cultures, inspiring swiftness in innovation. The winged horse has the capacity to touch the heavens.

Celtic Symbolism: Horse is a symbol of victory. In Irish mythology, a horse named Enbarr, which means "imagination," could run swiftly without touching the ground or water.

Cautionary Message: Do not hold the reins too tightly. Allow yourself to explore new terrains and consider where the winds of change are inviting you. As you embrace your newfound freedom, be mindful not to abandon your integrity, all that makes you uniquely you.

Moose

Traits: Moose are known for their size, measuring up to six feet tall and weighing about 1,000 pounds. The antlers of a male moose can be up to six feet long. Because of their height, they feed on leaves and shrubs in forested areas rather than grass. In the winter, they eat tree bark, twigs, and whatever is not covered in snow. Moose will become aggressive to protect themselves or their calves.

Archetypal Image: Moose is the gentle giant archetype, possessing great stature, strength, and power, while also being mild-natured and noble. Moose reminds us that power and humility can be a magnetic combination. Moose encourages us to be confident and bold but not to exert force over another.

Indigenous Symbolism: Moose represents enduring strength and stamina, both powerful and gentle. The Mi'kmaq people of Nova Scotia regard the albino moose as sacred and not to be hunted.[33]

Cautionary Message: Do not underestimate the power of humility. To be humble does not mean that your way is unimportant or incorrect. It simply means there are other ways.

Mountain Goat

Traits: Mountain goats are related to antelopes and gazelles. They are extraordinary climbers and can maneuver their way up near-vertical cliffsides in order to evade less sure-footed predators. They are also quite territorial and have been known to knock another mountain goat off a cliff. They roam in small groups and thrive in colder climates.

Archetypal Image: Mountain goat represents the explorer archetype, who is willing to climb to extraordinary heights and adapt to changing climates. Mountain goat reminds us to set clear boundaries to avoid misunderstandings. It encourages determination and persistence as we seek to overcome obstacles that stretch our resources.

Cautionary Message: If your focus is on being the greatest of all time, you might miss out on the ultimate climb—that is, to become the greatest version of your most authentic and joyous self.

Rabbit

Traits: Rabbits are known for their prolific reproductive habits. At just two or three months old, a rabbit is ready to start its own family. As they have many predators, they can run swiftly and for long periods. In the wild, rabbits can exist in extreme temperatures, creating systems of tunnels under the ground. They are social creatures and form large colonies.

Archetypal Image: Rabbit is often portrayed as the trickster archetype, lightheartedly deceitful and resourceful. Rabbit is also the outlaw archetype, stealing from gardens for its needs to be met and always on the run, evading capture. Rabbit reminds us to survive against all odds, that we are deserving to be here on this earth simply because we exist. Rabbit encourages us to be resourceful and abundant.

Indigenous Symbolism: Rabbit is a happy-go-lucky trickster and a symbol of fertility.

African Symbolism: Rabbit is portrayed as a clever trickster.

Eastern Symbolism: Rabbit is associated with gentleness and the energies of the moon.

Celtic Symbolism: Rabbit is mysterious and swift, possessing supernatural, shape-shifting powers and embodying energies of the moon and of Earth.

Cautionary Message: You cannot evade everything that provokes the sensation of fear. Recognize that fear often precedes growth and naturally arises with new opportunities or change. Remain grounded, ask for and accept support, and trust in the natural order of all things.

Snake

Traits: Though snakes have poor eyesight, they can sense heat, which alerts them to the presence of prey. Snakes smell with their tongue and breathe through their skin and mouth. They perceive their surroundings with the vibration of their jaws on the ground or in water.

Archetypal Image: While some teachings relate the snake to the sinful and evil trickster, the snake archetype represents wisdom, healing, and transformation in many cultures. Snake reminds us to tap into our inner resources by paying attention to our bodily sensations and all that we feel. Snake encourages us to regularly shed what is no longer essential to our growth and to readily embrace transitions.

Indigenous Symbolism: Snake is the guardian of great wisdom that can yield danger or healing.

African Symbolism: Snake is sent by the ancestors as a message of approval or warning, depending on the type of snake. In Benin, a country in West Africa, there is a sacred shrine known as the Temple of Pythons constructed as a tribute to the serpent deity named Dan. Pythons are revered as symbols of wisdom, good fortune, and peace.

Eastern Symbolism: The snake is symbolic of great power, water spirit, renewal, and transformation. Snake also represents the Kundalini energy that resides at the base of the spine that is ready to be mobilized to balance the body.

Celtic Symbolism: Snake represents wisdom, healing, and transformation.

Cautionary Message: As you shed what you no longer consider to be useful, be sure to honor all parts of your journey. Hold on to the essential parts of you.

Spider

Traits: Spiders are skilled engineers of highly organized webs made of silk secreted from their bodies. Their hairy feet prevent them from sticking to their own webs and allow them to walk on ceilings. Having eight legs allows spiders to escape predators and survive with fewer legs. Some spiders have eight eyes, allowing them to see in multiple directions, while others live in dark caves and have no eyes. Though solitary creatures, spiders communicate through pheromones and vibrations when it is time to mate and reproduce.

Archetypal Image: Spider is the creator archetype, masterful weaver of intricate designs. Spider invites us to continually bring new concepts into this physical reality. Spider recognizes infinite possibility amid uncertainty.

Indigenous Symbolism: In Hopi culture, Grandmother Spider connects the past to the future and carries the wonders of creation inside every web.[34]

African Symbolism: In the Akan tradition of West Africa, spider is a trickster god known for wit and creativity. The Mambila people of Nigeria and Cameroon practice spider divination, where decisions are made based on a spider's movements around cards and other objects.

Eastern Symbolism: Spider is revered for ingenuity and wisdom. Spiderwebs symbolize happiness and good fortune.

Celtic Symbolism: Spider is a weaver of destiny.

Cautionary Message: Do not become entangled in webs of comparison and envy. Your destiny lies in creating the best version of your life, not in comparing your accomplishments with those of others.

Turkey

Traits: Wild turkeys are known to be curious explorers, foraging the ground for food, alert and with keen hearing and excellent eyesight. They travel in flocks and communicate through distinct calls that help them reassemble when one of them has been lost. Together, they sun and preen their feathers to maintain their health, regulate their temperature, and rid themselves of parasites. At night, they know to roost in trees to avoid predators.

Archetypal Image: Turkey is the archetype of community and connection. Turkey encourages us to accompany each other, to explore the world around us, and to find ways to live together in harmony. Turkey reminds us of the abundance that exists in nature, our relationship to the sun, and to the solid ground we walk upon.

Indigenous Symbolism: Turkey feathers have been used in ceremony as symbols of abundance and pride. The Mashpee Wampanoag, "the people of first light," so called because they were first to see the sun in present-day Massachusetts and eastern Rhode Island, were some of the nations known for their feathered robes. Turkey is honored for its nobility and for its sacrifice as an important source of food.

Cautionary Message: Do not give from a place of emptiness, guilt, or expectation. Rest and restore to give from a place of abundance, a place that honors our sacred connectivity.

Turtle

Traits: Turtles have been around since the age of dinosaurs. They live incredibly long lives due to their ability to protect themselves from cell damage. A turtle's shell acts as a shield from predators. Turtles are solitary animals; they bask and migrate as a group not to socialize but to increase their chances of survival.

Archetypal Image: Turtle is the explorer archetype, having seen Earth through many ages. Turtle values independence, freedom, and connection to the land and the sea. Turtle reminds us to enjoy moments of solitude to deepen our self-awareness and to be able to think for ourselves.

Indigenous Symbolism: Turtle is the symbol of Mother Earth. In a Taino legend, a zemi, or deity known as Deminan Caracaracol, had a female turtle growing on his back. This turtle is said to be the origin of the human race.

African Symbolism: Turtle symbolizes fertility and protection. In the West African country of Senegal, the endangered African spurred tortoise is a symbol of fertility and longevity.[35]

Eastern Symbolism: Turtle is wise and holds within it the history of Earth and secrets of the universe. In Taoism, turtles are mediators between heaven and earth, reminding us of the interdependence of all nature. Korean monks practice "compassionate release" as a way of ensuring and respecting life.

Celtic Symbolism: Turtle represents grounded wisdom, longevity, and protection.

Cautionary Message: You are not meant to carry the world on your shoulders. Retreat into your inner sanctuary when necessary. Establish safe boundaries but do not withdraw completely into yourself.

PET MESSENGERS

Dreams of pets are often vivid and can involve varying degrees of emotion. You might dream of a living pet, a recently deceased pet, or a childhood pet. You might awaken to find that your room smells like the pet that is no longer with you. Your dreaming mind might provide you the opportunity to experience what it might feel like to hold your pet once again, to see them healthier than they were in their final days. These dreams enable us to see the power of love and connection that is shared with our faithful animal companions.

Logan was my first pet, a yellow Labrador retriever that we adopted in June 2007. He was then 14 months old, gentle, loyal, and well-trained. Aside from the fact that he was attracted to the muddiest parts of our neighborhood pond, he was so easy to love. He remained with us for 11 years. A few weeks after we said good-bye, I had the following dream.

Date: July 11, 2018
Day of Week: Wednesday
Time: 5:13 a.m.

TITLE OF DREAM/THEME: *Logan Swimming with Frogs*

PEOPLE/PLACES/THINGS: *Logan, pond, frogs*

FEELINGS/EMOTIONS: *(During or after waking) Sense of amazement and peace*

COLORS: *Clear*

SYMBOLS: *Water, frogs*

DETAILS: *I see Logan swimming in a large pond. The water is unbelievably clean and clear. I am amazed that I can see all the way to the bottom. Logan seems so happy. A multitude of frogs begin to appear all around him. He continues to swim with them. The scene changes and I can now see him and the frogs swimming underwater. I wake up.*

INSPIRED ACTION STEPS/CHANGES/DECISIONS: *Look up the symbolism for frogs.*

Even before learning that frogs were a symbol of rebirth and renewal, this vivid dream provided an incredible sense of peace. Water typically represents our emotions, but swimming is also something Logan loved to do. I was curious why my dreaming mind did not place him in the muddiest pond. I was also wondering how he might feel about my decision for us to get another dog right away, a new puppy this time. According to Dream Moods, an online dream dictionary, "To see calm, clear water in your dream means that you are in tune with your spirituality. It denotes serenity, peace of mind . . ."[36] Seeing Logan underwater showed me that he is now in a different realm than I was used to seeing him. His legs and hips were strong and flexible once again. He seemed content and at peace, as if to indicate that he was okay with our family having another loyal companion. In fact, it was the timing of his death that led to us having a puppy in our home just one week later, allowing us to experience joy and sadness side by side.

STEPS FOR ENGAGING WITH ANIMAL ARCHETYPES

1. Record the details of the dream and, if you so desire, give it a title.
2. Consider the emotions that you experienced in the dream or upon waking.
3. Consider which animal traits and/or symbolism most resonates with you.
4. Write, draw, paint, or use other creative expression to further engage the animal messenger.
5. Share your dream with at least one other person if you feel comfortable.

DREAM VISUALIZATION PRACTICE: AN ENCOUNTER WITH AN ANIMAL MESSENGER

Dreamscape: Sitting at the edge of a river, surrounded by mountains. An animal messenger appears on the opposite side of the river.

Objective(s): To observe and engage with an animal messenger. This could be a pet or wild animal. This practice can be done after an animal dream or as a meditative experience for self-exploration.

Visualization: Rest comfortably in this moment, here and now. Become aware of your breathing, this sacred breath of life. Breathe deeply, allowing the breath to nourish your entire body. Exhale deeply, surrendering to the peace of the present moment.

Breathe in, allowing your shoulders to relax even more as you begin to feel a greater sense of ease. Breathe out and surrender. Breathe in. Breathe out.

Imagine yourself sitting alone at the edge of a river surrounded my mountain peaks that extend to the clouds. Hear the rushing water that has made its way hundreds of miles down the mountains to where you now sit. Observe the water as it flows, making its way around stones of every shape and size. Notice the ripples that will continue to travel and find their way into other nearby brooks and streams.

Now, bring your attention to the opposite side of the river. Allow yourself to fully let go and just observe. See which animal wishes to come to you.

Continue breathing, letting go, surrendering to the moment as your animal messenger makes an appearance.

Will it emerge from the forest or approach from the air?

Is this messenger typically a solitary animal or did it lose its way from its flock or herd? Does it sit peacefully, observing its surroundings, or is it on high alert?

What strengths does this animal possess? Do they reflect qualities that you most need right now?

What message might this animal hold for you?

Thank this animal for its presence and for its messages.

When you have finished expressing your gratitude, bring your awareness back to your breath. Feel your feet on the floor once again and take note of any bodily sensations. Gently open your eyes and return to this present time and space, fully reinhabiting your body.

Embodiment: Record the details of this experience, including the messages that were revealed to you. Consider the qualities of the animal that was present to you. Which quality appeals to you most? How can you embody this quality in your current life experience?

Chapter 10

LUCID DREAM HEALING

"Once you stop fighting for the life you think you're supposed to have and start living the life you want, every-thing seems to fall into place." I recorded these words in one of my journals back in February 2001. I believe they were spoken by a guest on *The Oprah Winfrey Show*. Fast-forward to January 2008, one month after my sixth pregnancy loss, I reread these words in my journal and tore out the page, crumpled it up, and threw it into the trash. In that moment, I interpreted the words to mean that *I should stop trying to have another child*, which is not what I wanted to hear.

Four days after, while walking my dog, Logan, I noticed a paper on the ground with my handwriting. When I picked up the soiled paper, it was the same journal page I had thrown away. Somehow it had made its way out of the trash that was collected three days prior. I was curi-ous—I walked Logan multiple times a day but had not seen the paper until that moment. However, this day I was in a different emotional space and once again these words took on a different meaning. I was ready to admit that I had indeed been fighting, fighting to carry pain and hurt on my own because I thought I was supposed to. I had stopped living because I had not yet achieved the family that I had imagined. I had been waiting to take a family portrait because the family I had envisioned was not yet complete.

This was the same day I was scheduled to meet with a Franciscan nun named Irma. Reluctantly, I had agreed to see her at my mother-in-law's urging. The idea of sharing my innermost thoughts and feelings with a stranger was not something I wanted to do. Since I am not Catholic, I also had reservations about seeing a nun for guidance. As it turns out, she was exactly who I needed. She was the one who got me started on the path of healing, growth, and spiritual transformation. "Peace and harmony begin with self-knowledge," Irma shared. It seems I was finally ready to do whatever was needed to restore peace and harmony in my life.

The journey of self-knowledge is about becoming aware of all that we are. This awareness encourages us to embrace the stillness within ourselves that allows healing to emerge. With healing comes clarity. And with clarity, my dreams became more lucid. As a young child, I would frequently find myself awake in my dreams. I would know I was dreaming, but never did I experience the level of lucidity that I began to experience once I started my healing journey. This journey included reflective journaling rather than just documenting the events of my day, paying even closer attention to my dreams, developing a meditation practice, and allowing others to accompany me on this path of self-discovery.

August 29, 2012: *Though fully lucid, I am well aware that my body is asleep and that this is a dream. I am in Island Harbour near my aunt's house. The sun is just above the horizon. Where are all the fishing boats? There are absolutely no boats in the water, which is not typical at this beach. I see two people in the distance, a man and a woman I do not recognize. Now I'm standing on the sea rocks and my right foot slips. I end up scraping the inner part of my right leg, just above the ankle. I am surprised by the fact that I can feel pain though I know I'm dreaming. Still, it occurs to me that since this is a dream, I have nothing to fear. I will go into the water and swim out as far as possible in the wide-open sea. I feel a sense of excitement. Just as I enter the water, a tidal wave appears. The tidal wave lifts me out of the water and carries me a distance. It then deposits me inside my parents' home, which prompts me to wake.*

Almost immediately, I recognized that I was lucid dreaming. Awake in my dream, I could swim out into the deepest parts of the sea without fear of drowning. However, the memory of a childhood incident made its way into my dreamscape. I was 13 when I experienced a near drowning. My cousins and I had been volleying a ball in the water at a large family gathering. We often played in the sea without any adult supervision. This day, there were many adults present, so we ventured farther away from the shore. I didn't know it at the time, but this beach was known to have sudden drop-offs. I stepped back just a bit to reach the ball and found myself sinking. One of my cousins quickly came to my rescue, allowing me to escape physical injury. "You're fine," everyone reassured when I was safely onshore. Still, my active imagination continued to think of everything that could have happened, magnifying that moment so that I would never risk having that experience again. A place that had been my playground every summer for as long as I could remember then became the place I most feared.

Prompted by this dream, I used my early-morning meditation to visualize what it would be like to sit on the beach with my younger self. I imagined her telling me how frightened she had been at the thought of not being able to breathe, of no longer being with the people she loved, of no longer existing. My journal entry included a letter explaining that her brain had done exactly what it had been designed to do. Our brains are designed to protect us, to keep our bodies safe. I reminded her that in this moment, she is safe, and her continued uneasiness with diving in and swimming into the deeper parts of the ocean is completely understandable. I assured her that we could always enjoy the sea safely from the shore. A few weeks later, I had this non-lucid dream:

> September 19, 2012: *I am near the sea. I see a younger version of myself standing at the shoreline. She is facing the ocean; her back is toward me. She is barefooted, wearing an orange sundress. I watch from a distance, looking at her as she looks out at the ocean. I can hear the waves rolling in and out. I feel a sense of ease. Just as she turns to look at me, I wake up. It feels as though my childlike gaze upon the ocean has been restored in her and in me.*

These healing dreams were timely. In late October 2012, when my daughter was eight years old, our family took a trip to Anguilla. This was her first visit to the island. I was able to relax when at the ocean, and I allowed her to swim with her cousins and walk on the sea rocks. I even snapped a photo of her gazing out at the sea, just as I had done countless times when I had been her age. For the first time in years, I swam in the sea, and it was fun, even though I was still mindful to stay close to shore.

AWAKENING IN YOUR DREAM

To have a lucid dream is to be aware that you are dreaming while you are in a dream. Your body is physiologically in REM sleep, your brain is highly active, and your consciousness is awake. You know that your body is in bed, yet your senses attempt to tell you otherwise. At times, this state of awareness is immediately recognized. Other times, something out of the ordinary happens that clues you in to the fact that this must be a dream. For example, furniture might be arranged haphazardly in your home, or you may see something that could not possibly happen in waking life, such as a fish swimming in the sky. You might begin reading a brief note posted on your refrigerator only to find that the words keep changing before you get to the end, or you might perceive a level of clarity you've never experienced in waking life.

Being awake in your dream provides a unique opportunity to explore the nature of consciousness. Your dreaming mind is not simply mimicking your waking reality; it is making connections and creating a world of its own. Depending on the degree of lucidity, you can influence the content of your dreams. You can ask a question and receive a reliable response. The realization that you are dreaming can instantly transport you to another location. It can enable you to leap into the air and fly, or swim in the deepest parts of the ocean. Just about anything you can imagine, you can experience in your dreaming world. You might manifest a conversation with a loved one who can no longer be physically with you. You might decide to practice an instrument, engage in an athletic event, or other fun activity. You might use this opportunity to face an unresolved emotion, or you can receive guidance from your deepest wisdom.

Lucid dreaming allows you to understand how you perceive, how you think, and how your creative mind works in dream states. You realize that your perception can change in an instant. You can look at your hand, look away, then look back to find an additional finger. When it comes to how you think, your second thought could seemingly materialize before your first, allowing you to see how quickly your brain makes associations and connections. You can walk through walls and travel anywhere in the world—or beyond. The impossible becomes possible. If your mind conceives it, your dreaming mind can make it happen.

In the world of lucid dreaming, you can create alternate realities without losing touch with your current reality because you know that you are dreaming. But if you get overly excited about being lucid, the dream can immediately dissolve, and you'll wake up. For example, the sensation of awe I experienced in my lucid dream shared in Chapter 7 of being washed ashore; as soon as I heard myself say, "There's no way I could be here," I immediately woke up.

While the law of gravity often does not apply in lucid dreaming, other physical limitations or consequences can apply. In my tidal wave dream, I was made aware that my dream body could perceive pain when it encountered a sharp object. While I have no recollection of ever slipping on the sea rocks and getting hurt, it was likely something I thought about and managed to avoid in waking life.

When lucid dreaming, the dreamer is less able to avoid what arises in one's awareness. Similarly, what is hidden or dormant in the subconscious always makes its way to the surface.

There was no physical reason for me to experience pain in my leg. When I woke up, there were no scratches or bruises. I had no leg pain prior to or after this dream. Some lucid dreamers say that they have never experienced pain in their dreams, while others confirm that they have. Just as the sensation of cold can evoke a dream of being caught in an ice storm or the sound of a whirring fan can create a helicopter in your dream, physical pain experienced in waking life can be realized in both lucid and non-lucid dreams. On the other hand, some lucid dreamers with chronic pain report a reduction in the intensity of physical pain after a lucid dream experience. Take the following dream experiences of two of my patients, both who came to me as a result of having some sort of chronic pain.

J.H.'s Dream

For weeks now I've been having migraines—I would wake up with one just about every single day. Last night, I dreamed I was having a terrible migraine. The pain was so intense that I was crying uncontrollably. I looked over to my left and saw my grandmother standing at the foot of my bed. I knew right away that this was a dream. She came to the head of the bed and placed her hand on my forehead. I woke up this morning without a migraine. Go figure.

T.R.'s Dream

I deal with chronic back pain. I dreamed I was lying on what looked like a massage table, but it wasn't a place that was familiar to me. I noticed a window to my left and light was coming in. A woman came into the room. She said I could sit up now. When I sat up, my back was not hurting anymore. I bent over to touch my toes and I didn't feel any pain. When I woke up, though, my back was still hurting.

HONORING YOUR DEEPER WISDOM

It is essential to recognize that your deeper wisdom is the gatekeeper of your dreams. You could have a strong intention to have a particular dream experience, but if it does not serve your whole being or could be triggering, your deeper wisdom will not allow it. Although I felt consciously ready to face my fear of swimming into the deep, my innermost being chose to be protective of this vulnerable aspect of myself. This tidal wave dream helped me understand that I could not override unresolved emotions even in my dream states.

Your deeper wisdom is not simply a passive observer. It acts in accordance with your whole being, not just in service to your conscious mind. It has an in-depth understanding of your mind, your physical body, your intuitive body, and your emotional body. It knows all that you have ever experienced whether you consciously remember or not. Your deeper wisdom also holds an accurate account of everything that has been experienced by ancestors from generations long past. It provides clarity, not confusion. It seeks truth in a balanced and expansive way, rather than narrowed judgment or exaggeration. Your deeper wisdom connects you to the wisdom inherent in all other living beings. It connects you to a force of love, truth, and greater understanding.

A tidal wave first appeared as a dream sign soon after the loss of our baby Jade. While I was clearly immersed in grief, this tidal wave also seemed to reflect an aspect of my deeper self. As shared in my introduction, when I ran toward the sea in search of my daughter, the tidal wave gently lifted and carried me until I woke up in bed. There was a sense of clarity the morning after this dream. Though I had suffered a great loss, my thoughts were more focused on my two-year-old, who needed her mother. I was prepared to do everything I could to heal for her. Now whenever a tidal wave appears, I recognize it as a powerful symbol reorienting me toward healing and purpose. Similarly, in lucid dreams I allow myself to be lifted and carried. This is also how I live my waking life, surrendering to the deeper mysteries I cannot yet understand.

BECOMING LUCID

Becoming lucid is about seeing ourselves, our connections to one another, and how we are interwoven into the fabric of the much larger world around us more clearly. It is about recognizing the seeds of possibility that exist within uncertainty, the hope in the midst of hopelessness, the purpose in the midst of pain and heartache. Becoming lucid is about deciding to not give up in the middle of a difficult journey, to take charge of our lives and change direction when necessary. It is about making choices that align with who we are and all that we intend to be and do with our lives. Becoming lucid does not mean that we automatically become all-knowing and all-seeing. It means that we recognize our capacity to discern what would serve our highest expression, which ultimately leads us to where we can best serve.

Lucid and non-lucid dreams alike can reflect our level of self-awareness and our capacity for growth and transformation. Both types of dreaming can illuminate areas of our lives where healing is necessary. Both can reveal hidden bias, resentments, unmet needs, unresolved conflict, and unfulfilled waking dreams. Lucid dreams allow us to participate in our healing since we can recognize different aspects of ourselves in real time. Our most vulnerable self and our most confident and empowered self can take the form of dream characters. Being conscious in our dreams enables us to engage with these parts of ourselves more fully. We can hear what each part has to say, the parts of us that are affirming and the parts that are critical and sometimes self-loathing. We can address past experiences, present concerns, and worries about the future.

Josiah's Lucid Dream

I was sitting on a bench in my neighborhood with a group of people I didn't recognize, but it seemed that I knew them in my dream. The dream is taking place a few years into the future, and we were contemplating the state of our world. I was struggling to come up with a good solution for all of us and knew I needed to somehow find wisdom. I started levitating and hovered over the pond near the bench we were sitting on. I flew up to a tree and I noticed a floating book enveloped in golden glitter flying in front of me. I opened the book up to a random page and read the first sentence of a random paragraph. It said, "I know the answers you seek, for I too have opened my third eye." I immediately knew it was something important, so I got down from where I was and tried running back to my house to write down all the words so my waking self could find the truth. However, as I ran back to my house, the dream ended abruptly.

Since lucid dreaming most often occurs in longer REM cycles before we awaken, we can more easily recall the dream narrative. While we may not be able to hold on to every detail of the dream, the essential message comes through.

Lucidity in a dream can further enhance our creativity and problem-solving ability. During sleep, our brains can access knowledge and experiences that we may not easily recall in our more conscious states. We can ask questions of our dreaming mind and we can receive reliable answers. In a 2021 study published in *Current Biology*, researchers found that lucid dreamers were able to accurately communicate solutions to mathematical problems while they were asleep.[1] Using voluntary eye movements and facial muscle contractions, dreamers were able to answer yes-or-no questions and respond to other stimuli, allowing them to be interviewed while they were still asleep. One of the participants, a 19-year-old male, had only two lucid dreams prior to this study, indicating that this ability is not unique to experienced lucid dreamers. A 20-year-old participant with a diagnosis of narcolepsy was described as having "remarkable lucid-dreaming abilities." He was able to enter REM sleep one minute after falling asleep and signaled that he was lucid dreaming just five minutes into his dream. Not only does this research confirm the ability to solve problems while physiologically asleep but it also recognizes real-time communication that can occur between the waking and dream states.

DEVELOPING A LUCID DREAM PRACTICE

While becoming conscious in your dreams can happen spontaneously, lucidity can be practiced and developed. Renowned dream researchers like Stephen LaBerge and lucid dreaming teachers such as Charlie Morley and Clare Johnson have written extensively, sharing specific techniques to help dreamers have more lucid dreams. Here are three exercises that I have found useful, on knowing your dream signs, knowing your environment, and practicing your dream scenarios.

Exercise 1: Know Your Dream Signs

Knowing your dream signs helps you to know when you are dreaming. Once you have been recording your dreams for a while, you get to know what you most commonly dream about. Create a list of dream signs from your dream journal. A dream sign could be a relative in the Spirit realm, a place that you cannot easily go to in your current reality, or even a celebrity. If your ordinary dreams repeatedly feature a specific animal, you can develop the awareness that whenever you see this animal, there is a greater likelihood that you are dreaming. This awareness alone can trigger lucidity. Review your dream signs before bed. Once you recognize that you are dreaming, you can awaken more fully in your dreams.

Exercise 2: Know Your Environment

Another lucidity trigger is when you notice that a room is arranged differently than how you are accustomed to seeing it. Dreams will often reconstruct your home or other familiar environment with added features that will get your attention. Practice present-time awareness whenever you can to deepen this recognition. For example, while brushing your teeth, look around and notice the details around the sink, the floor, the window, the door; slowly scan the room and really notice your surroundings. Notice if any emotions arise within your body. The more you do this in your waking states, the more you develop your ability to suspect when you are dreaming.

Exercise 3: Practice Your Dream Scenarios

Once you know your dream signs and deepen your present-time awareness, practice creating your dreamscape as with dream incubation. Set the intention to see one or more of your dream signs. Right before falling asleep, picture a particular sign you would like to have show up in your dreams. If you would like to wake up in a specific destination, research that location, look at photos, and invite it into your dreams. If you could be anywhere in the world, where would you like to go? How adventurous do you want your dreamscape to be? Have fun with this exercise.

J.G.'s Dream

I once dreamed I was in an African savanna, hiding in the bushes, trying to avoid elephant poachers. I was looking for an opportunity to stop them. A poacher was one step ahead of me, and he pulled out his musket and fired it. I could feel death approaching, but I refused to give up hope on saving the elephants. I put my hands together as I shouted, "Kamehameha!" Kamehameha is the name of a ruler who was born in the Kohala Mountains of Hawaii. His name means "the very lonely one" or "the one set apart." My aura flared up and burned bright with intensity. A blue energy beam protruded from my palms and vaporized everything in front of me, and I knew it was finally over as the dream ended.

DREAM VISUALIZATION PRACTICE: JOURNEYING THROUGH SPACE, OBSERVING EARTH BELOW

Dreamscape: Safely floating in outer space among the stars, observing Earth below. Alternatively, you can imagine sitting in front of a movie screen, watching a recording of outer space.

Objective(s): To explore within the depths of your imagination what it might be like to observe Earth from outer space; to recognize the bigger picture of all that you are and your connection to a much larger universe

Visualization: This practice can be done seated or as you lie in bed.

Sit or lie comfortably in bed. Feel your mind relaxing, as images of the day begin to dissolve behind your closed eyes. Feel your muscles softening as your body becomes more and more relaxed. Breathe normally. Feel no expectations, just complete surrender into relaxation as you fall asleep.

Know that you are safe and that this experience can be whatever you want it to be.

Imagine waking up in a dream. You have the awareness that your physical body is safely asleep, but your dreaming body is weightless, floating miles above Earth, among an ocean of shimmering stars, of varying densities and brightness.

You might see yourself alone, floating through this dimly lit sky, or you might envision other dream bodies in the distance. Whatever you decide, know that you are never completely alone. You are always being guided.

Allow yourself to feel at home among these magnificent, twinkling lights.

Notice the empty spaces between the stars, appearing as darkness. Allow yourself to be carried through these empty spaces, weightless and uninhibited, as your consciousness explores this infinite universe.

What is contained in these stars is also contained within you. You and I are made of millions of particles, and all the empty spaces connect and unite us.

Now imagine yourself looking back on Earth, at our shared home. Notice that there is one continuous planet with varying landscapes but no dividing lines or obvious boundaries.

Whatever thoughts or emotions arise, allow them.

Notice the thin layer of protection that surrounds Earth. This thin layer of atmospheric protection allows Earth to exist as it is, allowing you and I to exist as we are.

Allow your consciousness to move closer and closer to Earth's atmosphere, where you can now see the interconnected oceans and landmasses. Imagine your dreaming body moving across the sky, allowing you to see the unique ecosystems, the mountains, rivers, vast deserts, cities and towns, oceans and seashores, islands—everything that makes up this extraordinary planet. This is your home. This is our shared home.

Now, imagine returning to your current reality, this moment in time and space. Your consciousness now returns to your physical body, allowing you to awaken.

Embodiment: When you are ready, open your eyes. As always, take a few minutes to fully reinhabit your body. As you journal about this experience, I invite you to consider these thoughts: From the vantage point of space, there are no clear-cut geopolitical boundaries, just one continuous living, breathing planet surrounded by a thin layer of atmospheric protection in an expansive universe. This is our home. She deserves our mindful awareness, our conservation, our care. What affects one, affects all. Can you feel the truth of these words within your body? What thoughts or feelings arise? What is one way that you can care for our planet?

Chapter 11

CHANGE YOUR DREAMS, CHANGE YOUR LIFE

Regardless of where you live on this planetary star, each time you drift into sleep, you have an experience that scientists cannot yet fully explain. For decades the prevailing theory has been that our nighttime dreams are the by-product of physiological processes resulting in random firings of neurons in the brain. Elders in many cultures would disagree with that theory. Some would say that dreams come from Source, God, Soul, Great Spirit, the Infinite, the divine within us, or from parallel universes, ancestral or karmic imprints. My grandmother believed that dreams provided guidance from a source of higher wisdom unless they were scary. Then she would say, "Child, did you forget to say your prayers last night?"

Prayer has been central to my journey. It has been a source of comfort, strength, and ever-flowing peace. One of the fertility specialists I saw had a sign in his office that caught my attention one day. It read, "Peace comes not because your prayer has been answered exactly as you prayed it but because you shifted your focus and the burden . . ."[1] The burden of broken dreams can cause us to question everything we have ever known. Recurring pregnancy and birth loss caused me to question everything about myself, including my faith. Still, with each disappointment I continued to prayerfully ask for guidance, paying close attention to the messages of my dreams and to the synchronicities that followed. This allowed me to see that our dreams, no matter where they come from, are more than just misfiring neurons in the brain.

> July 2, 2017: *"I have a gift for you,"* an unknown dream figure says to me. In the dark of the night, I cannot see his face clearly. He has a grandfatherly presence. He takes my hand in his and places "the gift" into the palm of my hand. When I look at my hand, it is closed. I awaken not knowing what the gift could be.

We were at Hampton Beach in New Hampshire when I had this dream. We made a spontaneous decision to take a weeklong vacation that coincided with someone else's last-minute cancellation, allowing us to secure a rental right on the beach. That was a gift, being able to walk the beach each morning at sunrise. This one day, I decided to walk the boardwalk, connecting all the little shops along the main street. I went alone. We had already been there a few days, but for the first time a sign for a tiny Tibetan store caught my attention. I went inside and ended up purchasing a few books and a meditation CD. I was about to leave when the clerk said to me, "Oh wait, I have a gift for you," echoing the words that were spoken in my dream. He did not take my hand in his as the dream figure had, but I did feel a wave of energy course through my body as he handed me a bookmark. It contained a message from the 14th Dalai Lama. It spoke of religious diversity and of love and compassion being an essential component in every religion. It reads, in part, "All religions share a common root, which is limitless compassion. They emphasize human improvement, love, respect for others, and compassion for the suffering of others."[2]

WHAT DON'T YOU ALREADY KNOW?

While dreams can confirm important life-altering decisions, they do not simply lead us to what we already believe or know. They require us to adopt a sense of humility, a quality of openness that allows us to have new experiences and gain a wider perspective. Though dreams are symbolic in nature, the synchronicities that follow in waking life point to there being some larger force at work. As soon as I was back to the apartment on the beach, I opened my journal to reread the details of my dream and to record the synchronicity with the Tibetan store. This was not the first incidence when someone unexpectedly used the same words that had been spoken to me in a dream. The message on the bookmark was already something I strongly believed. What, then, was this dream trying to show me? I turned the bookmark over and read, "Made in India by Tibetan refugees." I did not know anything about Tibet, so I imagined that this could be where the dream was pointing me.

Since dreams are of the unconscious, they guide us to uncover something that is not in our current awareness. They help us to express what we are not already expressing. This could be an unexpressed thought or emotion.

It could be a hidden or unexpressed talent or unrealized potential. Dreams open us up to the realization that sometimes the answers we seek are not the ones that we find. They often challenge us to grow beyond our current way of thinking. They can lead us in a direction we might be less inclined to consider. An example of this would be the unknown dream figure, the doctor who proclaimed that I would require surgery to survive my pregnancy. I was hoping for validation that I should reach out to the midwife who had seen me through my only successful pregnancy. Instead, I received a direct statement that did not align with what I wanted. There was no reason to suspect that I would require surgery during a pregnancy. Back then, I assumed my dreaming mind was overstating the fact that an obstetrician would be ideal in my case.

Dreams are persistent. If the message of a dream is urgent but not understood, it will be repeated in the form of a recurring dream. If it is ignored, it will return. If it is forgotten upon waking up, it will be come back again and again. A recurring dream could feature the exact dreamscape with similar characters, or the imagery could vary. However, the theme remains the same so that the message can be received. As mentioned in an earlier chapter, there are times when dreams evolve as we evolve. A dream's message may unfold over many years like my dream of the fish in the crib. It took almost 15 years for that message and my grandmother's interpretation to be understood. I suspect that this dream will continue to unfold as I continue to evolve.

DREAM YOGA AND SLEEP YOGA

Remaining open to the idea of learning something new is what led me to discover Tibetan dream and sleep yoga. The term *yoga* is a Sanskrit word most commonly translated to "yolk," recognizing our ability to become more aware and to connect with something beyond *the self*. Dream yoga and sleep yoga are spiritual practices that utilize lucid dreaming to explore the deeper aspects of our unconscious mind and connect to the larger reality that we are all a part of. Traditionally, these ancient practices are used by Buddhist practitioners to prepare themselves for the process of dying. These practices can also help us to live a fully awakened life.

In dream yoga, it is less about controlling the dream than it is about being conscious in your dreams and experiencing the limitless nature of the mind. As you become aware of how illusions and projections are created in the landscape of the mind, you begin to recognize the dreamlike quality of the external world—the impermanence of not only material things but also your emotional state and the challenges that you face in waking life. You become aware of how the environment can reflect what you feel. Or maybe the emotions you feel are the result of what is happening around you.

Dream yoga helps us observe and allow without judgment or expectation. We begin to recognize that darkness is not to be feared or avoided, but to be observed and explored. Likewise, the darkest moments of our lives are not intended to break us and cause undue suffering but to awaken us fully to our light—the light of awareness and the light of compassion for ourselves, for others, and for the world we live in. According to Tenzin Wangyal Rinpoche in *The Tibetan Yogas of Dream and Sleep*, dream yoga increases our capacity to "transform anger to love, hopelessness to hopefulness, what is wounded in us to what is healed and strong. We develop the ability to work skillfully with the situations in life and to be of aid to others. . . . Then we can change ordinary life into experiences of great beauty and meaningfulness, incorporating everything into the path."[3] As we do this, we begin to see that anything we experience can be transformed into greater purpose.

One dream yoga practice is to use the power of the imaginative mind to interact with and alter the appearance, shape, size, or quantity of any object in the dream. With intention, you can transform one flower into a field of flowers or a toy dragon into a real dragon right in the middle of your living room. You can transform yourself, becoming an eagle and experiencing a more expansive sense of freedom. You can become an oak tree and experience greater strength and stability. You can transform into a more fearless version of yourself and decide to choose life no matter how difficult that choice becomes.

Rinpoche's book also helped me to better understand a dream experience that began in childhood and continued into adulthood. I was about 12 when I first woke up in a dream where I experienced total darkness. I was completely aware, but there were no images, no awareness of the room I was in, no awareness of my sister in bed lying next to me, and no awareness of my physical body. I waited to see what would happen, but nothing did. I then tried with all my might to wake myself up. I tried to cry out, but again, nothing. I remember thinking that maybe I died in my sleep. I didn't know what else to think. What felt like hours later, I woke up with a clear memory of the experience. This continued to happen. Each time, I would have a similar response but knew that I would eventually wake up. I never knew how to explain this experience of "total darkness" to anyone else, so I kept it to myself.

This experience differs from my experience of sleep paralysis. With sleep paralysis I experience awareness of my body even though I am not able to move. I am aware of the room I am in even though I cannot open my eyes to see it. I am aware of my husband in bed next to me and when I manage at least to moan, he can hear me and wake me up. In reading Rinpoche's book and learning of sleep yoga, I realized how closely my experience resembles sleep yoga; as though I was on the edge of it but not able to experience it fully without proper understanding and guidance.

Sleep yoga is known to Buddhist practitioners as "sleep of clarity" or "clear light sleep." It is when the body is experiencing dreamless sleep—no images, only an emptiness that is filled with pure awareness. This emptiness is referred to as "the mother," while the light is referred to as "the son, *rigpa*, pure innate awareness."[4] When we experience this type of sleep, known as the inseparable nature of the mother and son, we experience the true nature of understanding. "Ignorance is compared to a dark room in which you sleep," Rinpoche explains. "Awareness is a lamp in that room. No matter how long the room has been dark, an hour or a million years, the moment the lamp of awareness is lit the entire room becomes luminous."[5]

Significant blood loss after losing my son, Jackson, made it necessary for me to remain sedated until I had received multiple transfusions. While others with near-death experiences have shared amazing interactions with angelic beings and of having pure awareness while they were unconscious, I had no recollection of images or visitations or anything else. I remained curious about the fact that I could recall just about every detail before losing consciousness, even my last thought, but then nothing else. I was told that my husband was not allowed to stay at my bedside because each time he did, my heart rate elevated too high, which indicated that I was aware of his presence. However, I had no memory of him being at my bedside. "Maybe you were off visiting your babies," one friend offered.

The curiosity about that experience arose again as I began writing this book in October 2020. My last thought before losing consciousness had been about my daughter. My prayer was simply that I needed to be here for her. It had been five days since I had seen her. The first thing she said in the presence of my husband was, "Mommy, I had a bad dream. I dreamed that you were in the hospital and that you died." She was five years old at the time. Days later, my mother-in-law shared that she was calling for me in her sleep, saying "Momma," the night I had been unconscious when no one knew until the next day what had happened.

One of my friends recommended hypnosis to try to recover any unconscious memories from that time. If I was meant to remember anything, I imagined it would surface in my dreams. One night I asked for a dream. My intention was to remember only if it would serve my highest expression. The next morning, I awoke from this dream.

Date: December 6, 2020
Day of Week: Sunday
Time: 4:12 a.m.

TITLE OF DREAM/THEME: *Clear Light*

PEOPLE/PLACES/THINGS: *Light*

FEELINGS/EMOTIONS: *(During or after waking) Peaceful awareness*

COLORS: *Clear*

SYMBOLS: *Light*

DETAILS: *I wake in my dream. There is awareness of light around me. There is no awareness of my body or where I am. I am in motion, moving steadily toward what at first appears to be a tiny spark of light. The spark becomes larger and brighter as I approach. It expands in front of me, around me, and now it contains me. There are no other thoughts in this awareness, just light. I wake up.*

I feel a sense of peace as I lie here, awake in this current reality. It occurs to me that I did not experience any discernable emotions while in the dream. There was no sense of awe or curiosity. My only focus was the light. As I try to further express what I've just experienced, it feels as though I was in an enclosed area at first, though I could not visualize any boundaries. It reminds me of when I'm looking through an otoscope into a patient's ear—visually it's an enclosed space, and I could see the tiny spark of light being reflected off the eardrum. As the light grew and became more expansive in my dream, it appeared to envelop the entire space, including me. It seemed like I was suspended in the light, but I did not have this thought while in the dream. I was without thought or emotion.

INSPIRED ACTION STEPS/CHANGES/DECISIONS: *The realization that sometimes there is no action, no step, no change, no decision to be made, just the awareness of what is. That is all.*

I now realize that while I did not experience angels on the other side, I did encounter angels on this side, in human form. Not only doctors and nurses but also a janitor in the ICU I will never forget. Every year, particularly around Thanksgiving season here in the United States, I send a quiet blessing to this man and his family. I can still hear his voice in my mind. "Well, you look better than you did yesterday," he had said. "Looks like you're gonna be okay." He was a grandfatherly figure, mopping the floors in my hospital room. I looked up to acknowledge him, managed a smile, but my eyes quickly fell back to my sheets. "You're gonna be okay," he said again. This time he stopped mopping and stood at the foot of my hospital bed as my eyes met with his. In that moment, I believed him. For the first time that day, it felt as though I would be okay. A stranger, who had no reason to care, was the voice I most needed to hear.

PRACTICING DREAM YOGA

Dream yoga depends on the ability to lucid dream. It is an advanced practice that ideally follows a specific sequence involving waking at two-hour intervals throughout the night. While I prefer to not have interrupted sleep, there have been nights when I have unintentionally awakened every two hours and was able to complete the sequence. I created the following outline to better understand the practice of dream yoga as discussed in *The Tibetan Yogas of Dream and Sleep.*[6]

With dream yoga, specific sleep postures are recommended. According to Tibetan tradition, the channel along the right side of the male body houses mostly negative emotions, while the channel on the left side of the female body does the same. For this reason, men are advised to sleep on their right side with their knees bent for stability, with their left arm resting along their left side. Women are advised to sleep on their left side, knees slightly bent with their right arm resting along the top of their side. Closing off the nostril on the side you are lying on is also recommended. These postures are believed to open the flow of wisdom.

THE MAIN DREAM YOGA PRACTICE (4 PARTS)

Part One

> **Objective(s):** To be an open channel. To generate peaceful dreams.
>
> **Time:** Around 10 P.M.
>
> **Body posture:** Men lying on their right side, women lying on their left side
>
> **Location of image/attention:** Throat center (throat chakra)
>
> **Image:** A red lotus flower with four petals with a crystalline Tibetan *A* at its center. If you practice drawing the letter, it will be helpful to reproduce mentally for this dream practice and others.

Instruction: While lying in the recommended body posture at bedtime, gently focus your awareness on the throat center. Visualize a red lotus flower with four petals at the throat center. In the center of the red lotus, there is a crystal that is shaped in the form of the Tibetan *A*. This crystalline *A* reflects a red light that radiates a peaceful glow. As you descend into sleep, imagine that your conscious awareness and your energetic body connects to and merges with this luminous red light. This will allow you to have peaceful dreams.

Part Two

Objective: To experience a sense of radiant clarity

Wake time: Approximately two hours after falling asleep (around midnight)

Body posture: Men lying on their right side, women lying on their left side

Breathing: Inhale and gently hold your breath as you lightly contract the perineal muscles in the pelvic floor, continuing to hold the breath just below the navel. After just a few moments, exhale, relaxing the pelvic muscles and then your entire body. This breathing pattern is to be repeated seven times.

Location of image/attention: Center of the brow (third eye chakra)

Image: A white ball of light

Instruction: After two hours of sleep, wake and perform the breathing exercise for seven repetitions. Then, place your attention in the center of your brow, where there is a rotating ball of white light. See and feel your consciousness and your energetic body connecting to and merging with this rotating ball of light. Feel yourself being absorbed into this light, keeping your mind clear and staying present while you fall asleep.

Part Three

Objective(s): To harness a sense of power, safety, security, and strength as you fall into sleep. To encourage light sleep and induce lucidity.

Wake time: Four hours after initially falling asleep (around 2 A.M.)

Body posture: Lying on your back with your head and shoulders elevated on a pillow; your hips are open with your legs slightly crossed at the ankles, so your knees fall to the sides.

Breathing: Bring your attention to your breath and maintain this awareness as you breathe deeply and gently for a cycle of 21 breaths.

Location of image/attention: The heart center in the middle of the chest (heart chakra)

Image: The Tibetan syllable *hung* is inscribed in black and radiates blackness.

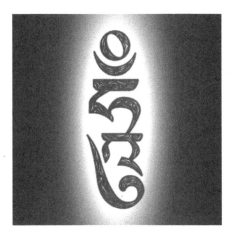

Instruction: After four hours of sleep, wake and assume the recommended body posture. Breathe gently and deeply for a cycle of 21 breaths. Visualize the Tibetan syllable for *hung* at the center of your chest. With intention, direct your energies to merge with the blackness that emerges from and through this symbol as you fall asleep.

Part Four

Objective(s): To bring awareness from the night into the day and from the day back to the night. To develop fearlessness.

Wake time: Two hours after your previous waking, but just before the light of dawn (around 4 A.M.)

Body posture: No specific posture

Breathing: Your natural rhythm

Point of focus: The area that sits behind the genital region (root chakra)

Image: A black sphere

Instruction: See your energetic body entering the black sphere and fusing with it. Allow the blackness to permeate all your senses as you fall asleep again. When you awake once more, enter your day with greater awareness. Carry this awareness throughout the entire day.

CHANGING THE DREAM

We each carry within us the capacity to create and destroy, to encourage and criticize, to be a voice of reason and one of despair. Our everyday thoughts and deeply held beliefs, conscious or subconscious, influence our day-to-day behaviors, habits, and choices. Our choices and actions influence our nighttime dreams. Dream yoga allows us to fully recognize the transformative power of our minds. If we can influence and change our dreams, transformation is also possible in our waking lives.

As Einstein is quoted, "We cannot solve our problems with the same level of thinking we used when we created them."[7] Our dreams allow us to come face-to-face with aspects of ourselves, but on a different level of consciousness. We can more easily recognize our destructive thoughts and our most critical voices. We hear more clearly the voices of our ancestors and our innermost self. Our dreams can show us how to live a difficult relationship with greater ease. We can then integrate these insights into our waking lives.

May 18, 2020: *We are in a familiar home, but there are noticeable differences such as the placement of furniture and appliances. She is a relative, but we haven't seen or spoken to each other in well over a year. We politely greet each other but exchange few words. I notice her blouse. The background is white with a black print of vines, flowers, and leaves. When she turns away from me, I notice a single red leaf in the lower right corner of her blouse. I awaken.*

The red leaf calls my attention. These words emerge: It reminds me of a time I felt envious of you. This envy came from a place of hurt and insecurity, feeling as though my body had failed me despite my best efforts, while you seemed to experience such ease with minimal effort—at least that is how it appeared to me. Now I recognize that we each have had our share of challenges that cannot be compared. For some reason, we are not meant to have the closeness I once envisioned. It has taken much time for me to accept this reality. Some days I still wish it could be different. Maybe someday it will be. When I move my awareness to my heart, I can easily recall other joyous moments we have shared . . . I envision you smiling, healthy, and safe. In this moment, I feel only gratitude. I send only love.

The guideposts for dream journaling and dream recall, shared in Chapter 1—awareness, compassion, trust, and sharing—are also relevant to changing our dreams and impacting our waking lives.

Awareness: It requires deeper awareness to see what is being reflected in our relationships, especially those that seem difficult. It requires awareness to choose again and again to be a healing presence rather than to perpetuate hurt. When we bring this level of awareness to our dreams, our dreams provide us with even deeper awareness. Through symbols and metaphor, we begin to see our roles in relationships more clearly.

Compassion: Changing the dream requires compassion for ourselves and for others. Compassion allows us to choose deep listening and empathy rather than trying to prove that the predominant way is the only way. Compassion recognizes the many facets and layers to who we are as individuals and as interconnected parts of a greater whole. In our dreams, our compassionate self can see from varied perspectives and make valuable connections we have yet to imagine.

Trust: The more we trust in the guidance that is available to us, the more we release our concept of time and timing. We recognize that change can happen spontaneously—maybe even overnight—or it can happen in such small increments that it remains invisible for much of the way. Trust enables us to begin where we are, using the tools and knowledge that we have while we await what comes next. As translated from the play *Faust*, by German writer Johann Wolfgang von Goethe, "Whatever you dream you can do, begin it. Boldness has genius, power, and magic in it. Begin it now."[8] Trust allows us to be bold in our living as we surrender to the unfolding.

Sharing: When we share our dreams, we hear them more clearly. This also allows others to participate in the message of the dream, and in the understanding of how the dream might change, evolve, and ultimately impact our lives.

BEGINNING A DREAM YOGA PRACTICE

Step One: Develop a Meditation Practice

Many lucid dreamers develop their ability to have regular lucid dreams in childhood or adolescence. A meditation practice deepens sensory awareness, allowing for greater clarity and longer, more stable periods of lucidity. Meditation also recalibrates the nervous system, bringing relaxation to the body and to an overactive mind so that you can readily fall asleep in a state of calm. Dream yoga practitioners recommend anywhere from 9 to 21 "purification" breaths as you prepare for sleep.

Step Two: Create a Sacred Sleep Environment and Invite Protection

In addition to ensuring your bedroom is dark, quiet, and at a cooler temperature that is conducive to sleeping (around 65 degrees Fahrenheit is recommended), prayerful intentions can also transform your room into a sacred space. Tibetan Dzogchen master Chögyal Namkhai Norbu suggests invoking protection by imagining loving beings surrounding you and remaining with you throughout the night as you sleep. I have been doing this at my grandmother's urging since I was a child.

Step Three: Bring Awareness to the Throat Center as You're Falling Asleep

As you drift asleep, imagine the red lotus flower attached to your throat. Softly focus on the emerging red light from the crystalline Tibetan A. Allow your consciousness and your energetic body to merge with this glowing light. This allows you to be an open channel, finding peace within yourself and allowing for peaceful dreams.

Step Four: Be Aware of the Dreamlike Quality of Waking Life

The practice of dream yoga is less about interpreting the messages of the dream and more about the awareness that this entire waking experience is *like* a dream. The more you acknowledge the dreamlike quality of your encounters, the more dreamlike experiences you will have throughout each day. For instance, you are standing outside when a dragonfly comes along, and you extend an open hand. It lands on your palm and stays there for quite some time. A few minutes later you realize that it is your grandfather's birthday and wonder if the dragonfly was letting you know that he is nearby. Or perhaps you are out walking your dog and you find a sealed envelope on a neighbor's lawn, with hearts all over, clearly the creation of a child. Days later, after a conversation with the child's mother, it turns out you're the unintended recipient of this envelope. You open it to find a card that reads, "Just for You" and a drawing that relates to a sign from a beloved teacher now in the realm of Spirit.

DREAM VISUALIZATION PRACTICE: RECEIVING A GIFT FROM A DREAM FIGURE

Dreamscape: Imagine falling asleep during a meditation and awakening in a dream. In this dream, you are sitting on a bench at the edge of a large pond, observing the changing landscape of autumn. Here you are visited by a dream figure who places a gift in your hands. This gift could be anything—a book, gemstone, pendant, object from childhood, or something that belonged to a loved one.

Objective(s): To practice the red lotus flower meditation that is used in dream yoga. To witness the creative and transformative power of your mind. To set the intention to receive a gift in an actual dream.

Visualization: I invite you to sit comfortably with an open heart and an open mind, your palms facing upward, indicating that you are ready to receive. Close your eyes or lower your gaze when ready.

Take a few slow, quiet breaths as you rest your awareness in the present moment. Continue breathing, finding a rhythm that is most comfortable for you.

Imagine being surrounded by pure white light. This light offers a sense of protection. Know that you are completely safe, that you are guarded, that you are protected. You may feel the presence of an ancestor or other benevolent being.

Breathe deeply.

Now see yourself lying in bed on your left side or on your right side.

Bring your awareness to your throat center as you imagine a red lotus flower attached to the center of your throat. It just sits there, upright. Though you are lying on your side, it remains in place.

Imagine there is a crystal in the middle of the red lotus flower, reflecting a soft, red light.

Imagine the energy of your energetic body flowing from all areas of your body, slowly moving toward this red light, merging with it.

Now imagine falling peacefully into sleep. You awaken in a dream where you are sitting on a bench near a large pond. Across the pond, there are rows of trees, their leaves are changing, ushering in a new season. Notice their shades of yellows, oranges, and reds. Delight in this colorful painting. Notice the cool, crisp air. Notice the fallen leaves at your feet, the ones that have already surrendered and await their return to the soil.

Imagine looking to your left as a dream figure—perhaps unknown, perhaps not—approaches and offers you a gift. Extend your hand to graciously receive this gift. The gift is gently placed into your hands.

Watch as your mind reveals this gift. Don't force anything. Just observe what happens. If you have difficulty visualizing this gift, what is the first thing that comes to mind? With your inner vision, see this gift. Observe its color, texture, size, and shape.

Be sure to thank your dream figure for this gift before they depart.

When you are ready, slowly bring your awareness back to your breath. Feel your feet on the floor. Take note of any bodily sensations. Gently open your eyes or raise your gaze as you fully reinhabit the present time and space.

Embodiment: If you wish, take a few moments to record details of this experience. What is the significance of this gift? How does it relate to what is occurring in your life? If you encounter this object or something similar in another dream or in waking life, record the synchronicity.

Chapter 12

OUR SHARED DREAM FOR COLLECTIVE HEALING

Years ago, I was given a ceramic candleholder depicting Christ's crucifixion that used to belong to my grandmother. There is a dove on each side, but one is broken. What is left now appears to be a butterfly. Since receiving this candleholder, whenever I am visited by a dove my thoughts immediately go to my grandmother. A particular series of dove sightings over the course of a week prompted me to share the experience with a friend. She messaged me back with a photo of a business card. Just moments before receiving my message, her home had been inspected by a company named Dovetail Home Inspection. "What do you think is your grandmother's message?" my friend asked. As I later contemplated the message of the dove and the butterfly, these words arose:

July 26, 2020: *My dear, brokenness does not diminish wholeness. The dove is still a dove, though she now appears as the image of a butterfly. The butterfly is also whole just as she is now; no mending required. See the beauty of the dove. See the beauty of the butterfly. Wherever she goes, whatever she becomes next, her essence will always be wholeness. See her in all her beauty.*

REMEMBERING OUR WHOLENESS

Our deepest wisdom is always guiding us toward wholeness. Our essence is wholeness. Wholeness does not mean that we never become ill, feel discouraged, or experience woundedness. Wholeness encompasses every aspect of being human, the cycles of birth and death, of disintegration and renewal. To be fully human is to be vulnerable. To open one's heart to love is to open to the heartache of loss and disappointment. To remain openhearted after prolonged illness or other adversity can be challenging. And yet it is the only way to truly experience the fullness, the significance, of life.

There is a story told by activist Bayo Akomolafe: A father who knows of his impending death says to his son, "Let's build a house together before I go." It takes years for this father and son to construct a house. Finally, their mission is complete, and it is beautiful.

"Our work is done, Father. We have achieved what we wanted."

"Not quite," the father says as he walks up to the house. With a hammer in hand, he proceeds to break through a wall, creating a giant hole.

"What are you doing?" his son yells. "We've spent years putting up these walls."

His father responds, "My son, the house isn't complete until it is broken. Now a passerby will notice the hole in the wall. And he will stop and ask what happened to your wall. You will invite him in, offer him tea, and tell him the story of your broken house. This is how you will become good neighbors."

The reality is that we connect more deeply with each other through pain and adversity. Tragedy, loss, injustice, broken dreams—they awaken us to our common humanity. Beneath the throes of grief lies our capacity to care more deeply, beyond our immediate family and neighbors. Time and time again, we have seen how persons and communities come together during or after a tragic circumstance.

Our capacity for love expands when our hearts break open, igniting and fueling purpose and compassion. We see this in someone who has known homelessness and now feels compelled to help others who are without a home. It is this expanding capacity that allows a young mother who conceived her firstborn because of sexual assault to come to accept her child regardless of how she came to be. Our capacity for love and compassion is what makes forgiveness possible and the unforgivable more bearable.

We are living in times when the prevailing perspective is that we are more disconnected than ever because of technology, politics, racism, classism, sexism, and every other painful divide. And yet these divides can encourage the formation of new connections and new communities that extend beyond geographical boundaries. Bonds based on shared beliefs and strong resolve create new alliances and fellowships that may not have otherwise existed. We see others more clearly when we understand their lived experiences. Technology allows us to see far and wide. Through the lens of compassion, we begin to recognize that we want the same things: to live in a society that is more harmonious and more just, a society that upholds the inherent worth and dignity of every person. Where we differ is how best to create such a society and how we might share in that responsibility. As Martin Luther King, Jr. once wrote from his jail cell in Birmingham, Alabama, "I am cognizant of the interrelatedness of all communities and states. . . . We are caught in an inescapable network of mutuality, tied in a single garment of destiny. Whatever affects one directly, affects all indirectly."[1]

This "single garment of destiny" is illustrated by a story that was published in *YES!* magazine in 2015. It is about an unlikely friendship between Jacqueline Suskin, a poet who viewed the redwood forest as sacred, and Neal Ewald, the senior vice president of a timber harvesting company known for its controversial logging practices, including the use of toxic herbicides. As the article explains, they met at a farmers market where Suskin would create poems upon request. After a first poem, Ewald reached out with another request for a poem to read as he and his family scattered his wife's ashes in the ocean. "When he met me, he felt he'd been led to me for a reason," Suskin writes. "I was to write this poem for his wife." It was after delivering the poem that she learned of Ewald's connection to the forest. "I was overwhelmed with the feeling that we could collaborate and create change." And that is exactly what happened. Suskin's poems brought healing to Ewald, and Ewald's willingness to understand and compromise saved the forest.[2]

As we share our innate gifts, we participate in the cycles of giving and receiving, not only with one another but with every forest, every tree, and every organism that graces Earth. This is how we remember that we are inherently whole. It is to recognize the wisdom of Dr. King's message when he said, "I can never be what I ought to be until you are what you ought to be, and you can never be what you ought to be until I am what I ought to be."[3] By Suskin being the poet that she was meant to be and Ewald being the businessman that he was meant to be, an entire forest continues to be. This is the interdependent nature of reality.

ALIGNING WITH OUR DIVINE NATURE

You may not know the full extent of your gifts until you embrace them and allow yourself to grow into them. It can be difficult to explain your deepest passions and your mystical experiences to others. Instead of seeking external validation or attempting to deny or demystify your experiences, allow yourself the space required to grow into them fully. Know that you will be brought into alignment with how, when, and where to best use these gifts in service to the world around you. I cannot promise you that the path will be straight and well-defined. However, once you decide to step onto this aligned path, you will receive guidance from a multitude of sources—some known, others unknown, some human, others not so human.

On October 24, 2021, I awoke from a dream of standing outside my grandmother's house. In the distance, off to the right, I could see my daughter looking for a cat that belongs to her cousin. I called out to her, "He is over here." I woke up from this dream to our dog, Summer, barking.

It was 1:47 A.M. I went to see why Summer was barking. There was a cat outside on our deck, sitting right at the glass sliding door, looking in. This gray-and-white-striped cat looked exactly like the one in my dream. It looked as though it was well cared for but as far as I know, it did not belong to any of our closest neighbors. It also had to travel a flight of 12 stairs to get to our deck, and for what purpose? What led it here at this hour? I could not hear this cat from our bedroom upstairs, with all the windows and doors closed plus a whirring fan in our room. Despite Summer's barking, the cat stayed until I went to the door. I could choose to believe that this was merely a coincidence, but I felt that it was an indication that my expanding consciousness somehow allowed me to sense the cat's presence in my sleep.

This experience served to remind me of dreams I had when I kept my grandmother's candleholder at my bedside. For an entire week, my dreams featured biblical scenes, many of them relating to the crucifixion. One morning I dreamed that I was the Apostle Andrew. I woke up from this dream just after 3 A.M. My heart was racing as connections to Andrew also flooded my mind. The church that my grandmother took me to as an infant was Saint Andrew's Anglican Church located in Island Harbour, Anguilla. When I was about 12, my childhood friend invited me to attend church with her and her family. We were living in Saint Thomas, US Virgin Islands, at the time. That church was Saint Andrew's Episcopal Church. Then in June 2007, a chance conversation in a grocery store with a woman I never saw again led me to another Saint Andrew's Episcopal Church about seven minutes from my home in central Massachusetts. Saint Andrew is also the saint associated with fishermen and with women who wish to become mothers.

As I sat up in bed, recalling the content of my dream and the connections to Andrew, an image of a man's face also formed in my mind. It was of an author named Gerry Gavin—though I knew of him, I did not know him personally. I got out of bed, went to my computer, and felt compelled to send Gerry a message telling him about my dream. We were connected on social media because our first books were self-published around the same time, in 2012, and with the same publishing service. They also had similar titles; his book was *Messages from Margaret* and mine *Messages from Within*. I had not yet read his book and we had no prior interactions. Gerry wrote back that he too had awakened several times after 3 A.M. from a dream of a woman and a little girl needing his help. This is when I learned that Margaret was not a wise sage but an angelic being that Gerry channeled. He offered to write to Margaret on my behalf and see what messages she held for me. Here is part of the message that Margaret sent for me.

> *My dear Kathleen . . . there is, within your heart . . . a brokenness, if you will, that is associated with the way you came into this world. Rape is an action that is taken by an aggressor who does so for him to feel more powerful . . . because at the root of the action is a feeling of not being powerful . . . or a victim of some other circumstance. This sense of powerlessness . . . which has at its root fear . . . was planted as a seed in your heart since it was the feeling that both your father and your mother held within them at the time of your conception.*
>
> *It is now a nondescript fear that you hold within your heart, and while it might lie dormant . . . whenever*

*you are confronted with issues of loss . . . whether per-
sonal or even things that you might see on the TV . . .
your heart triggers a fear response that quickens your
heartbeat and places your body into what some might
call the "fight or flight" reflex.*

*This is what is happening to your heart, and it
will continue in this manner unless you can utilize
some tools to help it to quiet itself. I will help you with
those today.*

*But first let me speak to the message that you
received about being Andrew. To say that you are
Andrew does not mean just that you were him in
another lifetime. It speaks to the fact that your soul . . .
the soul that still exists and will always exist . . . gave
part of its energy to this body named Kathleen and
another part of its energy to Andrew, and just as I have
mentioned in the book . . . since there is no real "time"
to speak of . . . Andrew and Kathleen are existing at
the same time. You are aware of that which you call
the "past" because your collective memory does not
record things until they have technically "happened"
in the ongoing expansion of the universe. To give you
an example . . . because much of your "memory" is
dependent on what you "see" with your eyes . . . you
have developed your sense of history from artifacts and
texts and through science you see things in the exploration of the stars that have happened in what you call
the past. But you have not yet developed the ability to
tap into what you call the future . . . Except in your
psychic abilities.*

*As to the fish . . . the fish symbolizes a creature
that can live within its environment by both going with
the flow and fighting the flow when it is crucial to its*

continued existence . . . It also breathes comfortably within its environment because it has learned how to process its own oxygen.

You are in the same type of situation. As spiritual beings you have come into forms that are much more limited than you are used to . . . and often . . . to live the life that feels correct to you, you find that you are often "swimming upstream" against great tides. But you adapt and you learn to use this body to breathe.

Spend more time focusing on your breath. Look at the upstream swim as just a part of your nature . . . just as the fish does.

Fish also appeared to you when you were pregnant because it was symbolic of a new life form, as well as that which gives life. To the fisherman of Jesus's time the fish was both their livelihood and their very life because a great deal of the land was hard to farm . . . and fish were plentiful. Fish came to be symbolic of life.

The metaphor of becoming "fishers of men" was very powerful because it was what the original apostles were being asked to do. But the plan that Jesus had in mind was for them to spread the word of the "divinity of man," showing how God was alive in every living thing.

I hope that this message will help you and that it will allow your heart to beat a bit slower as you have nothing to fear. You are protected and loved.

Your book by the way brings people back to the original message; become like children.

Go in peace and love,
Margaret

I was completing my second book, *Messages from Children . . . and What They Can Teach Grown-Ups*, so this part of Margaret's message was timely. This letter also served as a catalyst for me to consider the effects of unprocessed trauma from the time of conception as well as inherited trauma, which have been more widely discussed in recent years. We are shaped and programmed in our mother's womb and by all that our ancestors have experienced. We must remember that we also inherit many of their gifts. Our ancestors did not have the technology, books, scientific advances, and all that is available to us. Yet they valued their dreams and their connection to all of nature. It is not to idealize one way of being; it is to utilize the abundance of resources, conventional medicines, ancient remedies, and traditions that are available to us. There can never be a single approach to any problem.

To align with our divine nature is to recognize that there is so much more to who we are and everything we have ever lived. Each of us in our purest essence is a luminous soul, a spark of the divine with creative abilities. We create as we are created. We receive as we give. We empower as we become empowered. We honor all that we are when we walk through the sacred doorway of our dreams and when we choose to live this present embodiment with integrity, intention, and purpose. When we nurture, encourage, and allow life to emerge from us and through us, we invoke the gifts of our divine heritage.

JOURNALING EXERCISE: CONTINUING THE DREAM

We cannot erase the earlier chapters of our lives, but we do get to decide how the rest of our story will read. Everything that we experience, the families we are born into, the challenges, the opportunities, the people who come into our lives along the way, as well as the books that show up—it all weaves together this incredible web that beckons us to dream a new dream for our lives.

Pause and consider the threads in your life that have led you to where you are now, that have created the quilt of your present self. How are you being called to heal, create, and live a fully awakened life? What might the new dream for your life be? What kind of world do you desire to create and live in? Consider your planetary offering. How are you truly meant to serve in these phenomenal times?

DREAM MEDITATION: LET US MEET IN THE INFINITE FIELD OF COMPASSION AND HEALING

Dreamscape: As Rumi is quoted, "Out beyond ideas of wrongdoing and rightdoing there is a field. I'll meet you there."[4] I invite you to sit, stand, or lie down on this grassy field. You will be guided to see your out breath as an expansive light, able to transmit love and compassion, hope and strength, as we connect to a larger field of compassion and healing.

Objective(s): To bring compassion to ourselves, to our loved ones, to our world, or to a difficult situation

Visualization: Be mindful of your posture as you sit comfortably with your chest slightly lifted, allowing your shoulders to gently open. I invite you to position your palms facing upward on your lap or on your knees, helping you to maintain this open posture.

Close your eyes or lower your gaze and bring your awareness to your breath.

As you breathe in, imagine a revitalizing breath entering through the heart, allowing your lungs to expand fully. And as you exhale, imagine the breath being gently released back through your heart.

See yourself crossing a bridge that leads to an expansive open field where others have arrived before you. Find your place in this field. Imagine yourself walking to a spot that is reserved just for you. Stand if you wish, or sit on a chair or on the ground and feel your bare feet upon the grassy field. Feel the connection to the earth. This is your home.

Know that you are safe and supported, guided, and protected. Know that you are held in love's warm embrace.

Breathe in, deep into the belly, and breathe out.

Breathe in this nourishing breath that envelops your body, your heart, and mind as you experience a sense of ease and calm, a sense of love and compassion, hope and inner strength.

See your out breath as an expansive, luminous light, able to transmit love and compassion, hope and strength.

Imagine your breath merging with a larger field of compassion and healing. This larger presence knows your heart and the heart of all others. It can direct the energy of love and compassion to wherever it is needed, providing strength and peace, calm, courage, kindness, understanding, wherever it is needed, no matter how small or large the request.

As you breathe, allow the energy of this presence to return to your heart.

Feel the warmth of compassion being received through your breath. Feel it as it circulates throughout your body, throughout every system, every organ, in every tissue, in every cell, and to wherever you need it most. If possible, place your hand on this area and feel a luminous healing light penetrating it.

Notice whatever sensations arise in your body. Don't label them, simply notice.

Breathe in peace, breathe out peace.

Breathe in hope, breathe out gratitude.

Breathe in strength, breathe out courage.

In your mind's eye, visualize a person or persons in need of comfort or strength and offer these words: *May you know comfort. May you know strength. May you know that you are not alone.*

Imagine a wave of this compassion gently washing over them. Imagine them being comforted by it. Imagine that this breath brings them a sense of ease, that it brings them hope, that it brings them strength.

Now think of a challenging situation and allow the energy of compassion to freely flow to all involved.

Imagine yourself letting go of a specific outcome, not with the energy of defeat but with the energy of peaceful surrender. Allow for something beyond what you or others have yet to imagine.

May you know that you do not travel any path alone.
May you know peace within you and peace around you.

Allow this peace to occupy every cell in your body.
Breathe gently. Breathe easily.

Embodiment: Now take a moment to come back to your breath and reenter this present moment. Gently open your eyes or lift your gaze to fully return to the space that you are in. Reground yourself by feeling your connection to the floor, or perhaps place your hands on your belly or on your heart. Once again, may you know that you are connected to something greater. May you know that you are guided, guarded, and protected. Know that you are safe.

I encourage you to look for signs of planetary healing every day, knowing that we each can contribute to this shared dream of wholeness, and that you, too, can receive from this field of compassion whenever you need. It is available to each one of us simply because we exist in this world.

Remember, that we are each a unique expression of a masterfully woven whole. While no one person is responsible for healing all the suffering of the world, we can each contribute to its healing.

As for tonight, may you have a restful sleep. May your dreams be a source of guidance, inspiration, and healing. May you know peace. May you know love. And may we all be free.

CONCLUSION

As you continue to explore the wisdom of dreams, know that you do not have to do this alone. Everyone benefits from life-affirming connections and healing circles. Consider joining or starting a dream circle within your local area or participate in an online community where you can share and hear from other kindred hearts. I would be honored to accompany you in your dream explorations. It is also my greatest hope that you will decide to share these teachings with your children and grandchildren so that they, too, can realize that their deepest wisdom is always leading them toward wholeness, connection, and greater purpose. Let us dream. Let us live fully awakened. Let us create a society that recognizes the inherent worth and dignity of every person. It is up to all of us, not just a chosen few. Whatever we dream, we can create.

ENDNOTES

Introduction

1. Walker, Matthew P., et al., "Cognitive Flexibility across the Sleep-Wake Cycle: REM-Sleep Enhancement of Anagram Problem Solving," *Cognitive Brain Research* 14, no. 3 (November 2002): 317–324. https://www.sciencedirect.com/science/article/abs/pii/S0926641002001349.

Chapter 3: Understanding the Messages You Receive

1. Keller, Helen, *The Open Door* (New York: Doubleday, 1957).
2. (This quote was made popular by Martin Luther King Jr., but no clear evidence of when or where it was first spoken or written.)
3. Barks, Coleman, *The Soul of Rumi: A New Collection of Ecstatic Poems* (New York: HarperOne, 2001).

Chapter 4: Why We Hide, Run, Fall, and Fly

1. Laing, R.D., *The Facts of Life* (New York City: Pantheon Books,1976).
2. Rohr, Richard, *Falling Upward: A Spirituality for the Two Halves of Life* (Hoboken, NJ: Jossey-Bass, 2011).
3. King Jr., Martin Luther, "Keep Moving from This Mountain," address at Spelman College Museum (April 10, 1960): 10–11.
4. Allison, Sophia Nahli, "Revisiting the Legend of the Flying Africans," *New Yorker* (March 7, 2019). https://www.newyorker.com/culture/culture-desk/revisiting-the-legend-of-flying-africans.
5. Samples, Bob, *The Metaphoric Mind: A Celebration of Creative Consciousness* (Fawnskin, CA: Jalmar Press, 1993).

Chapter 5: Re-visioning "Nightmares"

1. Bell, Vaughan, "The Trippy State between Wakefulness and Sleep," *Atlantic* (April 20, 2016). https://www.theatlantic.com/science/archive/2016/04/deciphering-hypnagogia/478941/.

2. Morley, Charlie. "Experience Lucid Dreaming," Mindvalley (2021).

Chapter 6: *Dream Play* and Excavating Your Innate Gifts

1. (Attributed to Albert Einstein, but traced to Darryl Anka/Bashar https://quoteinvestigator.com/2012/05/16/everything-energy/#.)

2. Jackson-Buckley, Bridgitte, "Eliot Cowan: The Healing Wisdom of Plants," *BJBuckley* (December 17, 2018). https://www.bjbuckley.com/post/eliot-cowan-the-healing-wisdom-of-plants.

3. Redmond, Layne, "Priestesses of the Sacred Sound," *When the Drummers Were Women: A Spiritual History of Rhythm* (Brattleboro, VT: Echo Point Books & Media, 2018).

4. Ruhr-University Bochum, "How Playing the Drums Changes the Brain," ScienceDaily (December 9, 2019). https://www.sciencedaily.com/releases/2019/12/191209110513.htm.

5. R., Rory, et al., "Jose Aldo, the Beatles of MMA: Indisputable Greatness vs Loud Casual Consumption," Thread Head Media (December 26, 2021). https://threadheadmedia.com/mma/jose-aldo-the-beatles-of-mma.

6. Stumbrys, Tadas, et al., "Effectiveness of Motor Practice in Lucid Dreams: A Comparison with Physical and Mental Practice," *Journal of Sports Sciences* 34, no. 1 (2016): 27–34. https://doi.org/10.1080/02640414.2015.1030342.

7. PRH International, *André Rochais – Founder of PRH*, English translation (Altona, MB: D.W. Friesen, 1994): 63.

8. Zhang, Wenzhu, et al., "Synergistic Effects of Edible Plants with Light Environment on the Emotion and Sleep of Humans in Long-Duration Isolated Environment," *Life Sciences in Space Research* 24 (February 2020): 42–49. https://doi.org/10.1016/j.lssr.2019.11.003.

Chapter 7: A Sea of Ordinary and "Big" Dreams

1. Kennedy, John F., Remarks at the Dinner for the America's Cup Crews (September 14, 1962). https://www.jfklibrary.org/archives/other-resources/john-f-kennedy-speeches/americas-cup-dinner-19620914.

2. Foulkes, David, *Children's Dreaming and the Development of Consciousness* (Cambridge, MA: Harvard University Press, 2002).

3. Campbell, Jean, "Dealing with Precognitive Dreamer Guilt," *Electric Dreams* 8, no. 12 (San Francisco: DreamGate, 2001).

4. Cherry, Kendra. "Coping with the Fear of the Ocean," Verywell Mind (August 7, 2020). https://www.verywellmind.com/ thalassophobia-fear-of-the-ocean-4692301.

5. Loken, Erik K., et al., "The Structure of Genetic and Environmental Risk Factors for Fears and Phobias," *Psychological Medicine* 44, no. 11 (January 2014). https://www.ncbi.nlm.nih. gov/pmc/articles/PMC4079768/.

6. Aceto, Michael, and Jeffrey P. Williams, *Contact Englishes of the Eastern Caribbean* (Amsterdam: John Benjamins, 2003). https:// benjamins.com/catalog/veaw.g30.

Chapter 8: Dream Visitors, Known and Unknown

1. Myss, Caroline, *Intimate Conversations with the Divine: Prayer, Guidance, and Grace* (Carlsbad, CA: Hay House Publishing, 2021): 95.

Chapter 9: Engaging with Animal Archetypes

1. "Coyote, the Trickster," OCNews, Okanagan College (June 2, 2020). https://www.okanagan.bc.ca/story/coyote-the-trickster#s.

2. "Ancient Egyptian Jackal Figurine," Harvard Museums of Science & Culture, Harvard University. https://hmsc.harvard.edu/ ancient-egyptian-jackal-figurine.

3. van Huis, Arnold, "Cultural Significance of Lepidoptera in sub-Saharan Africa," *Journal of Ethnobiology and Ethnomedicine* 15, no. 26 (June 13, 2019). https://www.ncbi.nlm.nih.gov/pmc/articles/ PMC6567547/.

4. Deme, Mariam Konaté, *Heroism and the Supernatural in the African Epic* (New York: Routledge, 2010).

5. Olivera, Alejandro, Center for Biological Diversity (April 2018). https://www.biologicaldiversity.org/programs/international/mex- ico/pdfs/English-Top-10-Endangered-Mexico.pdf.

6. "The Story of Our Name," Leopard (February 8, 2022). https:// leopard.voyage/story-of-our-name-leopard/.

7. "Wolves in Native American Culture," American Wolves (June 3, 2020). https://americanwolves.com/blogs/wolf-stories/ wolves-in-native-american-culture#First_Sub_Point_3.

8. Mark, Joshua J., "Anubis," World History Encyclopedia (July 25, 2016). https://www.worldhistory.org/Anubis/.

9. McKee, Timothy Brian, "Great Blue Herons of Richland County: In Time and Timelessness," Richland Source (October 20, 2018). https://www.richlandsource.com/area_history/great-blue-herons- of-richland-county-in-time-and-timelessness/article_ad337016- d132-11e8-b9b3-2794977470b2.html.

10. Sherrard, Melissa, "Symbols of the Choctaw Indian Tribe," *Synonym* (June 30, 2020). https://classroom.synonym.com/ symbols-of-the-choctaw-indian-tribe-12083274.html.

11. "National Symbols," Embassy of the Republic of Indonesia (Washington, DC, 2017). https://www.embassyofindonesia.org/ national-symbols/.

12. "Birds - African Folklore," Wildlife Campus, African Folklore Course. http://www.wildlifecampus.com/Help/PDF/Folklore_Birds. pdf.

13. Ebersole, Rene, "Inside the Strange World of the Illicit Hummingbird Love Charm Trade," *National Geographic* (April 21, 2018). https://www.nationalgeographic.com/animals/article/ wildlife-watch-illegal-hummingbird-trade-love-charm-mexico-witchcraft.

14. Pennisi, Elizabeth, "Ravens—Like Humans and Apes—Can Plan for the Future," *Science* (July 13, 2017). https://www.science.org/ content/article/ravens-humans-and-apes-can-plan-future.

15. Sams, Jamie, and David Carson, "Dolphin," *Medicine Cards* (New York, St. Martin's Press: 1999): 196–199.

16. "We Are All Salmon People," Columbia River Inter-Tribal Fish Commission (January 31, 2022). https://critfc.org/salmon-culture/ we-are-all-salmon-people/.

17. "Why Is the Galjoen South Africa's National Fish Anyway? Here's Everything You Need to Know about This Part of Our Heritage," Two Oceans Aquarium, Waterfront, South Africa. https://www. aquarium.co.za/blog/entry/why-is-the-galjoen-south-africas-na-tional-fish-anyway-heres-everything-you.

18. "Spotlight On: Frogs," Stonington Gallery (Seattle: April 16, 2021). https://stoningtongallery.com/exhibit/spotlight-on-frogs/.

19. "The Cultural Significance of Whales in Hawaii," Go Hawaii (May 21, 2019). https://www.gohawaii.com/ the-cultural-significance-of-whales-in-hawaii.

20. McLean, Kim, and Devon O'Day, *Paws to Reflect: 365 Daily Devotions for the Animal Lover's Soul* (Nashville, TN: Abingdon Press, 2012).

21. "Whales in Mythology: History and Other Interesting Facts," Whale Facts (October 2, 2021) https://www.whalefacts.org/ whales-in-mythology/.

22. Christiansen, Paul, "Whale Worship: Exploring the Role of Whales in Vietnam's Coastal Lore," Saigoneer (April 10, 2018). https://saigoneer.com/saigon-culture/13047-whale-worship-exploring-the-role-of-whales-in-vietnam-s-coastal-lore.

23. Stepanek, Mattie J.T., *Journey through Heartsongs* (Alexandria, VA: VSP Books, 2001).

24. Gonzales, Patrisia, "Ant Medicine: A Narrative Ecology," *Chicana/ Latina Studies*, 1, no. 2, Mujeres Activas en Letras y Cambio Social (2012): 82–93. https://www.jstor.org/stable/23345343.

25. Ferre, Lux, "Ants in African Mythology," Occult World (August 3, 2017). https://occult-world.com/ants-african-mythology/.

26. "The Parable of Ants," *Economic Times*. https://economictimes.indiatimes.com/opinion/vedanta/the-parable-of-ants/articleshow/20546915.cms?from=mdr.

27. "The Native Meaning of . . . Symbology, Myths and Legends," My Mondo Trading. https://www.mymondotrading.com/native-meanings-symbology-myths-legends.

28. "Nandi Bear," DinoAnimals.com (November 11, 2020). https://dinoanimals.com/animals/nandi-bear/.

29. Russell, Deborah, "Legend of the White Deer," Authors Den. http://www.authorsden.com/categories/story_top.asp?catid=71&id=18862.

30. Diegor, Diane, "African Deer Guide: Meet the Barbary Stag (Africa's Only Deer)," Storyteller Travel (October 7, 2021). https://storyteller.travel/african-deer/.

31. "Engakuji Temple Kamakura," Japan Experience. https://www.japan-experience.com/all-about-japan/kamakura/temples-shrines/engakuji-temple-kamakura.

32. "The Wild Horses of the Namib," Namibia Tourism Board. https://namibiatourism.com.na/blog/The-Wild-Horses-of-the-Namib.

33. Al-Khatib, Talal, "'Spirit Moose' and Other Sacred Animals," Seeker, (October 11, 2013). https://www.seeker.com/spirit-moose-and-other-sacred-animals-1767943144.html.

34. "The Spider Woman," American Museum of Natural History. https://www.amnh.org/exhibitions/totems-to-turquoise/native-american-cosmology.

35. "African Spurred Tortoise," Lincoln Park Zoo (Manitowoc, WI). https://www.manitowoc.org/857/African-Spurred-Tortoise.

36. "Water," Dream Moods Dictionary. http://www.dreammoods.com/dreamdictionary/w.htm.

Chapter 10: Lucid Dream Healing

1. Konkoly, Karen R., et al, "Real-Time Dialogue between Experimenters and Dreamers during REM Sleep," *Current Biology* 31, no. 7 (April 12, 2021): 1417–1427.e6. https://www.sciencedirect.com/science/article/pii/S0960982221000592.

Chapter 11: Change Your Dreams, Change Your Life

1. Parkening, Christopher, and Kathy Tyers, *Grace Like a River* (Carol Stream, IL: Tyndale House Publishers, 2006).

2. His Holiness the 14th Dalai Lama, Tenzin Gyatso, *Toward a True Kinship of Faiths: How the World's Religions Can Come Together* (New York: Harmony Books, 2010).

3. Rinpoche, Tenzin Wangyal, *The Tibetan Yogas of Dream and Sleep*, ed. Mark Dahlby (Ithaca, NY: Snow Lion 1998): 138–139.

4. Rinpoche, *Tibetan Yogas*, 146.

5. Ibid.

6. Rinpoche, *Tibetan Yogas*, 104–118.

7. "Atomic Education Urged by Einstein: Scientist in Plea for $200,000 to Promote New Type of Essential Thinking," *New York Times* (May 25, 1946). https://timesmachine.nytimes.com/timesm achine/1946/05/25/100998236.html.

8. Corelli, Marie, "The Spirit of Work," *The Queen's Carol: An Anthology of Poems, Stories, Essays, Drawings, and Music by British Authors, Artists and Composers* (London: The Daily Mail, 1905): 31. https://books.google.com/ books?id=RkBAAAAAYAAJ&q=%22or+dream%22.

Chapter 12: Our Shared Dream for Collective Healing

1. King Jr., Martin Luther, National Urban League. https://nul.org/ news/letter-birmingham-jail.

2. Suskin, Jacqueline, "One Poem that Saved a Forest," *YES!* magazine (July 21, 2015). https://www.yesmagazine.org/issue/ make-right/2015/07/21/one-poem-that-saved-a-forest.

3. King Jr., Martin Luther, National Urban League. https://nul.org/ news/letter-birmingham-jail.

4. *The Essential Rumi*, trans. Coleman Barks (New York: HarperOne, 2004): 36.

ACKNOWLEDGMENTS

I offer my deepest gratitude to all those who participated in birthing this book: God, the loving presence that continues to guide me and open doors beyond what I imagined; Anna Cooperberg, my editor at Hay House, for your insight and commitment to ensuring clarity of my message; the entire Hay House family, especially Reid Tracy, Melody Guy, and Lisa Cheng, for your guidance in the early stages of this book; Gabby Bernstein, for these inspiring words: "If you want to really understand something, write about it; if you want to master it, teach it"; Kelly Notaras of KN Literary Arts, for your generosity with our first meeting, your expertise, and incredible team, especially Heidi McKye and Jennifer Bonessi; my chiropractic patients and wellness clients, for your trust in permitting me to share your dreams and healing experiences; Gail Van Kleeck, my writing companion, fellow author, and dear friend, for providing a nurturing space and the gift of your presence; the Hay House Writer's Community, for your enthusiasm, supportive feedback and inspiring voices; my family and circles of friends, near and far, who listen to my dreams and share yours with me; my ancestors, known and unknown, for accompanying me on this infinite path. I love you, eternally.

ABOUT THE
AUTHOR

Kathleen Webster O'Malley serves as a health and wellness practitioner, combining more than 20 years of chiropractic with other healing modalities that emphasize alignment to the body's inherent wisdom. A dream enthusiast since childhood, she encourages her patients and wellness clients to look to their dreams as a source of guidance, inspiration and healing. She is a 2020 recipient of the Visioneers Personal Achievement Award for her contributions to community wellbeing as a health practitioner, inspiring author and mentor to teens and young women. The Visioneers is a global community of change-makers.

Kathleen grew up in the Caribbean, among three island nations: Saint Martin—Sint Maarten, Anguilla and Saint Thomas. She currently makes her home in central Massachusetts with her husband, daughter and their dog, Summer. **www.kathleenomalleymessages.com**

Hay House Titles of Related Interest

YOU CAN HEAL YOUR LIFE, the movie,
starring Louise Hay & Friends
(available as an online streaming video)
www.hayhouse.com/louise-movie

THE SHIFT, the movie,
starring Dr. Wayne W. Dyer
(available as an online streaming video)
www.hayhouse.com/the-shift-movie

***

DREAM GUIDANCE: Connecting to the Soul Through Dream Incubation, by Machiel Klerk

DREAMING THROUGH DARKNESS: Shine Light into the Shadow to Live the Life of Your Dreams, by Charlie Morley

THE HIDDEN POWER OF DREAMS: The Mysterious World of Dreams Revealed, by Denise Linn

LUCID DREAMING MADE EASY: A Beginner's Guide to Waking Up in Your Dreams, by Charlie Morley

THE SHAMAN'S DREAM ORACLE: A 64-Card Deck and Guidebook, by Alberto Villoldo and Colette Baron-Reid

All of the above are available at www.hayhouse.co.uk

***

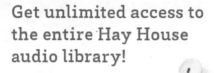
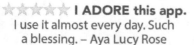

HAY HOUSE
Online Video Courses

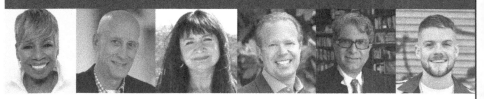

Your journey to a better life starts with figuring out which path is best for you. Hay House Online Courses provide guidance in mental and physical health, personal finance, telling your unique story, and so much more!

LEARN HOW TO:

- choose your words and actions wisely so you can tap into life's magic

- clear the energy in yourself and your environments for improved clarity, peace, and joy

- forgive, visualize, and trust in order to create a life of authenticity and abundance

- manifest lifelong health by improving nutrition, reducing stress, improving sleep, and more

- create your own unique angelic communication toolkit to help you to receive clear messages for yourself and others

- use the creative power of the quantum realm to create health and well-being

To find the guide for your journey,
visit www.HayHouseU.com.

HAY HOUSE
online learning